VITAMIN BEAUTY

Unleashing Your Glow With Vitamins Over Makeup

Samson Da Costa

Self Published

CONTENTS

AN INTRODUCTION TO THE WORLD OF VITAMINS

Have you wondered why your parents made you eat carrots? Why does sunbathing feel so good? The secret to our bodies' flawless operation is vitamins, small yet powerful chemicals.

This book covers four vitamins your body needs to survive. Imagine them as your body's VIPs: A, C, D, E vitamins. Each has its own ability, from night vision to converting sunshine into strong bones.

Fun Facts Box: Polish scientist Casimir Funk invented "vitamin" in 1912. He combined "vita" (life) and "amine" (a chemical) because he assumed all vitamins were amines. Despite being inaccurate, the name stayed!

Let's discuss why these four are so unique before we get into great detail on each vitamin. Unlike many other nutrients, your body cannot synthesize these vitamins from scratch—that is, except for vitamin D, but that is a bright tale we will come to later! You must receive them from either food or pills.

You might be wondering: there are lots of vitamins out there, so why focus on just these four? Well, these vitamins are like the foundation of a house - they support everything else. They're involved in crucial processes like:

- Keeping your immune system strong (imagine your body's personal security team)

- Maintaining healthy skin and eyes

- Protecting your cells from damage

- Building strong bones

- Healing wounds

- And so much more!

Unbelievably, many of us lack enough of these vital vitamins even in an age of plenty. Our contemporary way of life sometimes works against us: we spend more time indoors than we did years ago (goodbye, vitamin D from sunshine). We consume more processed meals, therefore farewell natural vitamins. And our hectic schedules often lead us to prefer convenience above diet.

Still, relax! This book will offer you easy, doable methods to receive these vitamins without radically altering your way of life. You don't have to spend a fortune on vitamins or start living like a health expert.

Let's first discuss something you have most likely seen but might not quite understand: nutrition labels before we get into great depth on any vitamin. On food containers, those enigmatic percentages and figures really tell a fascinating tale.

A label's "Daily Value" or "DV" indicates how much

of your daily vitamin needs that food supplies. The drawback is that these figures are averages; your age, gender, lifestyle, and even your location might affect your unique demands.

[Pro Tip: A 2,000-calorie diet is the basis for food label daily value %. Eat more or less than that, and your vitamin requirements may vary.]

Let us first get right to the fundamentals. A vitamin is like a small key opening vital operations in your body. Unlike carbs, proteins, and fats, you only need small amounts; nevertheless, these little amounts make a big effect.

[Except vitamin D, your body cannot create vitamins, so they are known as "essential". You have to receive them from either food or pills.]

Vitamins come in two main types: fat-soluble and water-soluble. Our fantastic four are split between these families:

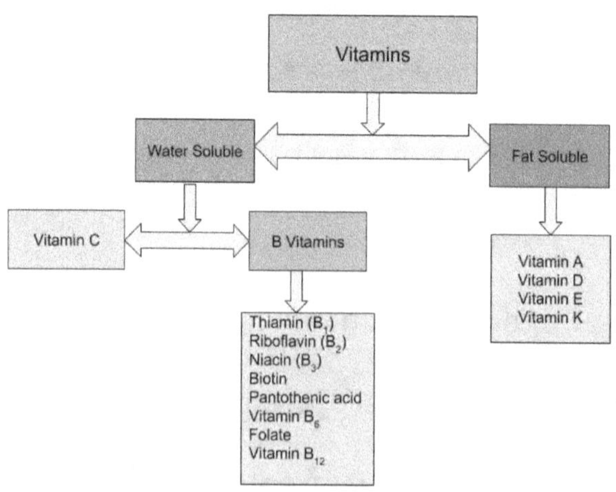

Stored in the body's fat cells, fat-soluble vitamins like vitamins A, D, E, and K can stay there for weeks or even months. Consumed alongside good fats, which improve their bioavailability, they are most absorbed. On the other hand, water-soluble vitamins —such as vitamin C—do not store well in the body; extra levels are eliminated through urine. To keep sufficient amounts, water-soluble vitamins must thus be routinely replaced from food.

The background of vitamin discovery is intriguing. People knew for millennia that some meals helped to avoid illnesses, but they were unsure about why. Citrus fruits stopped scurvy, sailors knew. Parents recognized that children grew robust with cod liver oil. Still, the scientific underwriting of it was unknown.

Scientists started separating and comprehending

vitamins not until the early 1900s. Every discovery addressed a unique medical riddle that had perplexed people for millennia.

Today's vitamin challenges are different from those of the past. We're not dealing with severe deficiencies like scurvy anymore. Instead, we face new challenges:

-Processed foods lacking natural vitamins

-Soil depletion affecting food nutrient content

-Busy lifestyles affecting eating habits

-Less sun exposure than ever before

Fascinatingly, vitamins cooperate better when taken together. For instance, vitamin D aids in calcium absorption; vitamin K ensures that calcium finds its proper location—that of your bones. Vitamin E performs better in presence of vitamin C.

"Should I grab supplements?" This could be the most often asked vitamin question of the modern era. Though the solution is not straightforward, here is the broad rule:

First food; second, supplements. Consider vitamins as backup vocalists; they are excellent help, but unless your doctor advises differently, they shouldn't be the primary act.

As you become older, your vitamin demands alter. Your body seems to be a car running on several fuels mixed in different ways at different phases.

Childhood: Great demands for development
Teenagers: More demands for personal growth

Adults: Degression of maintenance

Seniors: Many times require extra D and B12.

[Fundamental Knowledge: Not one-size-fits-all are vitamin requirements. They change with age, gender, lifestyle, and health issues.]

Deficit of vitamins vary according on where you live. While Americans could battle vitamin D insufficiency from indoor life, other areas deal with distinct issues:

Vitamin A insufficiency in Southeast Asia

Northern Europe: Deficiency of vitamin D

Many underdeveloped areas: Several shortages

Let's discuss how our food has evolved since we all live in this planet. Apple of today differs from that of your grandmother's apple. Longer storage durations, modern agricultural methods, and transportation have changed the vitamin count in our meals.

The positive news is More variation exists here than it has ever done. In your neighborhood supermarket are an orange from Spain, kale from California, and nuts from Brazil. Your secret weapon for acquiring sufficient vitamins is this diversity.

[Essential Fact: After one year of storage, a fresh apple can lose up to 75% of its vitamin C content.]

Your kitchen isn't just a place to prepare food - it's your vitamin preservation headquarters. How you store and cook your food can make a huge difference:

-Steaming preserves more vitamins than boiling

-Fresh-frozen vegetables often have more vitamins than "fresh" ones that traveled long distances

-Cutting fruits and vegetables right before eating preserves vitamin content

Nature has a remarkable way of providing the vitamins we need throughout the year, with seasonal foods aligning perfectly with our nutritional requirements. In the summer, we find light fruits rich in vitamin C, which help maintain hydration. As fall arrives, orange vegetables packed with vitamin A support our immune systems. During winter, root crops provide a valuable source of stored vitamins, keeping us nourished during colder months. Finally, spring brings fresh greens that are abundant in revitalizing vitamins, helping to rejuvenate our bodies after winter.

Your body's vitamin demands vary greatly depending on your lifestyle and everyday activities, just as various automobiles demand varied degrees of maintenance and fuel dependent on their use. Consider an athlete's body as a high-performance race vehicle; the higher physical demands, continual muscle repair, and higher energy requirements mean they need a more robust supply of vitamins to assist recovery and sustain top performance. Office workers, on the other hand, deal with their own dietary issues even if they are not straining their bodies to athletic levels. Long hours spent indoors under artificial lighting produce a particular demand for additional vitamin D, which we usually acquire via sunshine exposure. For pregnant women, whose bodies are essentially creating a new life, the situation is much different. Their vitamin demands vary generally to meet their own needs as well as those of their growing child, much as a car with a high load needs more gasoline and upkeep. Another special group are smokers, whose bodies suffer more oxidative stress from tobacco use and hence require more vitamin C to help to offset this extra strain.

Your body's shifting vitamin demands depending on your unique lifestyle and situation should be acknowledged and responded to, much as you wouldn't put ordinary fuel in a race vehicle or overlook the particular maintenance needs of a heavy-duty truck. These different demands emphasize the significance of realizing that vitamin consumption is not one-size-fits-all; your particular needs are as different as your daily schedule and living environment.

When it comes to vitamin levels, your body is a highly smart communicator that sends several signals to let you know if you're receiving enough. Consider these signals as your body's own health surveillance system, continuously offering comments on your dietary situation. Your vitamin levels will probably be appropriate and you will probably find a regular flow of energy throughout the day without the extreme highs and lows associated with inadequate diet. Your skin will show good vitamin levels by keeping its natural resilience and healthy radiance. Clear vision under different light levels, especially the seamless change from bright to dark surroundings, points especially to good vitamin A levels especially. Your body's natural healing abilities is another encouraging indicator; when cuts, scratches, or other small injuries heal within predicted times, it usually indicates that your vitamin levels are supporting your body's repair mechanisms. Your body does, however, also clearly alert you when vitamin levels can be low.

Here's something many people don't realize - stress affects how your body uses vitamins. During stressful times, your body burns through certain vitamins faster, especially vitamin C.

You don't need a degree in nutrition to shop smart for vitamins. Here's your simple guide:

-Color matters: Different colors mean different vitamins

-Fresh isn't always best: Frozen can be better

-Local when possible: Less travel time means more vitamins

-Whole foods over processed: Nature packages vitamins best

Eating for vitamins doesn't have to break the bank. Some of the most vitamin-rich foods are actually quite affordable:

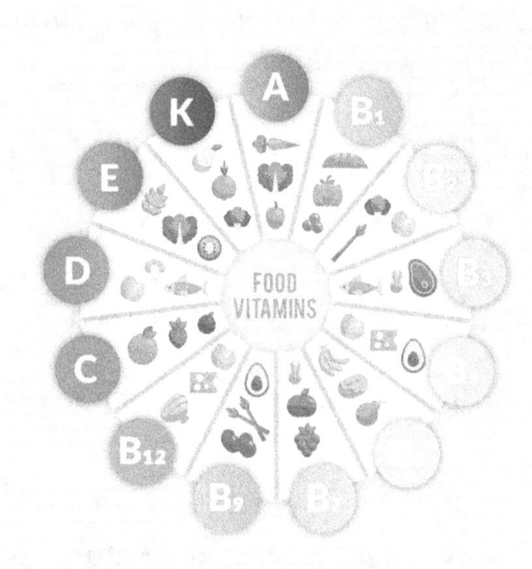

In the coming chapters, we'll dive deep into each of our four essential vitamins. You'll learn:

-Why each one matters

-Best food sources

-How to know if you're getting enough

-Common myths and facts

-Practical tips for daily life

Remember this before we get further into each vitamin: good nutrition is not about perfection. Mostly of the time, it's about making wise decisions. See this book as your helpful guide rather than a rigid rulebook. Use what suits you and expand over time.

ΔΔΔ

SEE CLEARLY WITH VITAMIN A

It's amazing how dark-colored cats can stand out so clearly, even in low light. Although we humans lack some natural ability, vitamin A is our night vision aid. Quite awesome, right? Though that's only the beginning of its powers, this superstar vitamin is your eyes' buddy.

Think of vitamin A like a master key in your body. It unlocks several important functions:

-Helps you see in dim light

-Keeps your skin healthy and glowing

-Supports your immune system

-Helps kids grow properly

-Maintains the health of your organs

And here's something fascinating: your body can store vitamin A for months, tucking it away in your liver like a squirrel storing nuts for winter.

Vitamin A has 2 forms:

1 Preformed Vitamin A (Retinol):

-Ready to use, no assembly required

-Found in animal products

-Your body's preferred form

2 Provitamin A (Beta Carotene):

-Needs conversion by your body

-Found in colorful vegetables

-Can't overdose on this form

[Important Note: Your body is smart! It converts only as much beta carotene to vitamin A as it needs. That's why you can eat all the carrots you want without worry.]

How much vitamin A do you need? It depends on who you are:

In adults:

-Men: 900 mcg

-Women: 700 mcg

-Pregnant women: 770 mcg

-Breastfeeding moms: 1,300 mcg

[Real Talk: These numbers might seem confusing, but here's what matters - eating one sweet potato or a large handful of spinach gets you there!]

Let's discuss how vitamin A supports eyeight. Special cells called rods and cones abound within your eyes. Like microscopic cameras, they capture light and convey images to your brain. Vitamin A keeps these cells in good functioning order.

Without enough vitamin A, objects appear dull and hazy, particularly at night, like attempting to capture pictures with a camera running low on batteries.

Let's investigate where in your daily meals vitamin

A lurks. Nature has two great cuisines with this vitamin. First, there are the contributions of the animal kingdom: eggs, milk, cheese, and fish where vitamin A is readily available. Consider them as your body's "fast food," quick and simple for your vitamin A intake. Though it's not everyone's favorite, liver is the unquestionably champion of vitamin A concentration. One plate of beef liver has many days worth!

Orange and yellow vegetables are like vitamin A in disguise - they contain beta carotene, which your body converts into vitamin A. Sweet potatoes, carrots, and butternut squash lead this vibrant parade. Surprisingly good sources are dark green veggies like kale and spinach; their green chlorophyll just covers the orange beta carotene hidden behind.

[Food Fact: One medium sweet potato supplies more than 100% of your daily vitamin A requirements!]

Mother Nature made it simple for us to get vitamin A; just search the vegetable sections for orange, yellow, and dark green items. Consider it as nature's traffic signal system: these hues indicate "go" for vitamin A. This is important because beta carotene content increases with depth in color. A dark orange sweet potato thus holds more vitamin A potential than a pale carrot.

Still, don't base meal decisions on its hue by itself. Some vitamin A superstars present unexpected packaging. For example, the brilliant yellow yolks of eggs have great vitamin A power. Furthermore, white milk is a consistent supplier of this essential vitamin even if it does not show its cards.

Your body's handling of vitamin A is very amazing; it's like having a savings account. Eating more than you need causes your body to save the surplus in your liver for later use. On your body's side, this is quite wise thinking; it's getting ready for periods when vitamin A may be limited.

However, there is a drawback. Your body need some fat for appropriate absorption of vitamin A. It's as though one needs a key to open a door. This is why eating your salad with some olive oil or having your carrots with some butter is not only delicious but also wise diet!

Your body has clever ways of telling you when it needs more vitamin A. The most obvious sign is trouble seeing at night - like when your eyes take longer to adjust when you walk into a dark room. Think of it as your body's check engine light.

Other signs include:

-Dry, rough skin (like sandpaper)

-Frequent colds and infections

-Dry eyes that feel scratchy

-Small bumps on the backs of your arms

-Delayed wound healing

Remember though, these signs could mean other things too, so don't jump to conclusions.

Like many wonderful things in life, vitamin A calls for balance. Though both too little and too much are issues. The wonderful news is if fruits and vegetables provide your vitamin A, you are in good shape; your body is clever enough to convert just what it requires from beta carotene.

The only genuine risk comes from supplements or consistent consumption of liver. Unless your doctor advises differently, it is therefore generally advisable to obtain your vitamin A from a range of foods rather than pills.

[Safety Note: Since too much vitamin A might harm the growing fetus, pregnant women should especially exercise great caution with vitamin A supplements. Generally speaking, food sources are safe.]

Within your retina, deep down is a remarkable mechanism converting vitamin A into sight. Vitamin A molecules change form when light strikes particular proteins known as opsins, set off a series of messages to your brain. From brilliant sunsets to faint shadows, this split-second change lets you see everything.

Vitamin A acts like a cellular telephone system, helping different cells in your body talk to each other. It carries messages that tell cells when to grow, when to specialize, and when to stop multiplying. This communication network is crucial for:

-Cancer prevention

-Embryonic development

-Tissue repair

-Hormone production

Programmes for vitamin A supplementation save millions of children's life all over every year. This vitamin is very important in underdeveloped nations in avoiding childhood blindness and lowering illness mortality including that of the measles. Among public health initiatives, the World Health Organization ranks vitamin A supplementation as among the most reasonably priced ones.

Several modern factors affect our vitamin A intake and absorption:

-Soil depletion reducing nutrient content in vegetables

-Air pollution blocking UV rays needed for beta-carotene synthesis in plants

-Modern farming practices affecting nutrient density

-Food transportation and storage reducing vitamin content

Different seasons bring different vitamin A needs and sources:

-Spring: Fresh greens and early vegetables

-Summer: Bright colored fruits and vegetables

-Fall: Orange squashes and pumpkins

-Winter: Root vegetables and stored produce

Understanding these cycles helps plan year-round nutrition.

In our digital age, vitamin A's role in eye health becomes increasingly important. Extended screen time can strain the vitamin A-dependent parts of your vision. Research shows that adequate vitamin A intake becomes crucial for:

-Blue light protection

-Screen fatigue recovery

-Eye moisture maintenance

-Visual stamina

Vitamin A intake is largely influenced by cultural eating habits. Fish oils and seaweed provide much of the vitamin A Japanese people consume. African people depend on palm oil and vibrantly colored root crops. Mediterranean eating calls for orange fruits and lush greens. Knowing these trends allows one to value the variety of sources of vitamin A.

Climate change affects vitamin A availability in surprising ways:

-Rising CO2 levels may reduce nutrient density in plants

-Changing rainfall patterns affect crop yields

-Temperature shifts impact vegetable growing seasons

-Extreme weather events disrupt food distribution

Beyond nutrition, vitamin A has applications in:

-Cosmetic manufacturing

-Food preservation

-Animal feed production

-Biotechnology research

All things considered, vitamin A is among the most adaptable nutrients available from nature; it serves several purposes in everyday bodily operations. Thanks to vitamin A's function in vision, you wake up and open your eyes; from then on, this nutrient never stops working—that is, from the moment you wake up and open your eyes to immune system support helps against infections throughout the day. It comes in two primary forms, according what we now know: the convertible form found in colored plants (beta-carotene) and the ready-to-use version found in animal goods (retinol). Whether our daily needs call for a plant-based diet or a mixed eating pattern, this dual-source approach offers us lots of choices.

The beauty of vitamin A is found in its storage capacity; your liver functions as a vitamin A savings account, accumulating extra for times when most needed. When foods high in vitamin A were rare, this clever biological mechanism enabled our predecessors to live through seasons. These days, it enables us to keep consistent levels even in cases when our meals are not flawless daily. A balanced diet heavy in colorful vegetables and certain animal products can easily meet your daily needs of 900 mcg (men) and 700 mcg (women).

As we have discovered, vitamin A has an amazing résumé of physiological activities. Especially in low light, you see it helps produce the light-sensitive proteins required for eyesight. Consider it as your own night vision engineer, continuously preserving and fixing the adaptation of your eye to darkness. Beyond eyesight, vitamin A supports your immune system's front-line defenses, helps create and preserve organ linings, supports appropriate growth and development, and aids in cell communication all across your body.

One cannot stress the worldwide influence of vitamin

A. Programmes for vitamin A supplementation keep saving millions of lives in underdeveloped nations. Its ability to counteract the consequences of our digital lifestyle, especially in terms of eye health, becomes even more crucial in the current society. A population that is well-nourished and has enough vitamin A access demonstrates much reduced rates of childhood death and improved general public health results.

Nature gives us enough from orange and yellow veggies, dark leafy greens, orange fruits, and animal sources including eggs and dairy. Scientific developments are helping to solve current issues such soil depletion, climate change, and altering agricultural systems, even while they may influence vitamin A availability in our diets. From better storage techniques to biofortified foods, we are discovering fresh approaches to guarantee everyone gets access to this vital mineral.

Remember that balance is important as we wrap up our vitamin A narrative; more isn't always better and dietary sources are often safer than pills. Consider your basic approach for obtaining sufficient vitamin A as consuming a variety of colors. Whether your breakfast is an egg, sweet potato, or a fresh carrot, you are feeding your body's demand for this vital vitamin. Maintaining foods high in vitamin A in your daily diet is not only about seeing better but also about living better, staying healthier, and supporting your body's amazing everyday operations in our modern society of processed foods and hectic schedules.

[Final Note: Although no one vitamin operates alone, vitamin A prepares several vital physiological processes. Remember that these nutrients cooperate like instruments in an orchestra to produce the symphony of well health as we advance to investigate vitamin C.]

△△△

MEET VITAMIN C– THE DAILY HERO

Imagine having a superhero that must show up every single day to keep you healthy—vitamin C. Unlike its fat-soluble cousins (such as vitamins A and D), vitamin C is like that buddy who never stays overnight; your body cannot store it for long and hence you need a fresh supply every day. Your body uses this essential vitamin in so many different ways that researchers are continuously finding fresh ones. From strengthening your immune system to assisting in collagen production, from combating free radicals to facilitating iron absorption, vitamin C is your body's best multitasker.

Along with guinea pigs, fruit bats, and certain primates, humans belong to a very exclusive club: we are among the few creatures unable to synthesize our own vitamin C. Every other animal generates it within their liver. For example, a goat may get up to 13,000mg of vitamin C daily—that is, around 170 oranges!

Consider vitamin C as your body's master builder. Its principal responsibility is Creating collagen: the protein maintaining everything in harmony. Your blood vessels require it to be strong and flexible; your skin needs it to remain firm and young; your joints need it to remain mobile. Vitamin C is there with its hard helmet on, supervising the building project, every time you heal from a cut, develop new skin, or mend any tissue damage. It also helps you to keep your teeth, bones, and cartilage. Actually, vitamin C is quite important for healing; so, doctors sometimes give patients suffering from accidents or surgery additional dosages.

[Note: Your body creates around one to two grammes of new collagen daily from vitamin C; this is like bit by bit building a small new you! This collagen formation would stop without vitamin C.]

See your body as a busy metropolis and free radicals

as little troublemakers rushing about wreaking havoc on DNA, destroying cells, and generally producing anarchy that could lead to aging and disease. Now enter vitamin C, the top security agent in your city! Acting as a potent antioxidant, this helps your body's defenses to neutralize troublemakers before they can inflict major harm. But it doesn't operate alone; vitamin C forms a complex defensive system with other antioxidants like vitamin E.

Let's dissect your vitamin C requirements so you won't lose yourself in a numerical jungle. Though some people require more, the average adult needs between 75 and 90 milligrams daily—that is around one big orange. Smokes require an additional 35mg as their body utilizes vitamin C quicker than others;

it's as though their cells are racing a marathon while everyone else is just walking. About 85mg is needed by pregnant women; nursing mothers need 120mg. Athletes, under pressure leaders, and those with illnesses might all require even more. The good news is that, unlike certain vitamins, vitamin C is somewhat difficult to overdo. Your body just gets rid of what it doesn't need, but too much might cause you a fairly urgent desire to use the toilet!

Forget the idea that just oranges are the vitamin C superstars. Nature has incorporated this vitamin into a brilliant range of foods. Particularly the red ones, bell peppers really have more vitamin C than oranges —that is, they are like oranges that got upgraded. Guavas are total champs; Kiwis are little vitamin C bombs. Even veggies with great vitamin C power are Brussels sprouts and broccoli. Surprisingly, potatoes —which we usually write off as simple starch bombs —actually help us consume far more vitamin C just by virtue of their frequency of use.

Your body uses vitamin C as a kid burns through their phone battery when you're worried. Whether it's a job deadline, a relationship issue, or even vigorous exercise, your adrenal glands burn vitamin C to generate stress hormones in trying circumstances. Though it's your body's emergency reaction mechanism, it need vitamin C as fuel. This helps to explain why you could become ill following a particularly demanding period: your immune system needs vitamin C most of which has been depleted.

Like that high-maintenance companion who is quite worth the work, vitamin C is It's sensitive to heat, light, and air, hence your cooking and storage techniques really count. If kept at room temperature, cut veggies can lose major amounts of vitamin C in a few hours. Cooking can also lower vitamin C concentration; but, there's a trick: rapid cooking techniques like stir-frying or steaming maintain more vitamins than long, sluggish cooking techniques.

Vitamin C is your buddy for your skin as much as it is for your interior wellness. Beauty businesses did not include vitamin C to their products haphazardly; this vitamin is essential for maintaining young, firm, and bright skin. It fights UV damage, can even help lighten dark spots, and generates collagen. Consider vitamin

C as your skin's own photographer; it will make you appear great in every picture!

Vitamin C is like a backstage support crew for athletes and fitness buffs. It lowers inflammation, aids in muscle damage repair following workouts, and could even assist with exercise-induced asthma. Certain studies indicate it might help ease pain in muscles following demanding exercises. It's like having a personal recovery assistant guiding you toward speedier post-training session bounce back.

Our current way of living poses special vitamin C problems. Our vitamin C demands can be raised by air pollution, smoking—even secondhand, stress, and certain drugs. Many times lacking in vitamin

C, processed foods cause a discrepancy between our requirement and what we obtain.

Although severe vitamin C deficiency—scurvy—is unusual in industrialized nations, moderate insufficiency is shockingly frequent. Studies indicate, especially in low-income regions, up to 15% of individuals could not consume enough vitamin C. Consider it as a concealed hunger, not strong enough to induce scurvy but sufficient to affect general health and well-being.

Time to debunk some vitamin C fallacies! No, megadoses won't stop colds (but enough vitamin C might shorten and milder). And even if most vitamin C pills are safe, more isn't usually better. Recent studies indicate it might benefit heart health as well as aid with anything from cancer prevention. Certain studies even look at its function in aging and brain health. Vitamin C reveals fresh abilities exactly as any good superhero would, right when we believe we know everything about it!

Nature offers a wonderful means of supplying exactly what we need, when we need it. Citrus fruits abound in vitamin C precisely as chilly season arrives. Winter comes Consider it: mandarins, grapefruits, and oranges all peak in cold months, as if nature's own immune-boosting prescription. With fresh greens and early berries, spring sweeps in with antioxidants when our systems are ready for regeneration. Summer offers a rainbow of fruits and vegetables, with additional vitamin C protection when we spend more time in the sun. Fall stocks us for winter by include robust veggies like bell peppers and Brussels sprouts.

This natural cycle is not random; it's much like nature's well scheduled vitamin C distribution mechanism. Understanding this cycle, our predecessors built their diets around seasonal availability. While most foods exist year-round today, eating seasonally still makes sense since it's when nutrients are at their best and costs are often lowest.

[Seasonal Tip: Since frozen fruits and vegetables are generally packed at peak ripeness, they are great sources of vitamin C when fresh choices are few or costly!

Vitamin C would be the most traveled upon if vitamins had passports! Travel surprisingly boosts our requirement for vitamin C. Flying dries us and exposes us to recycled air and plenty of viruses. While unfamiliar meals and surroundings tax our immune system, jet lag throws off our daily schedules. Smart tourists carry dried fruits, cherry tomatoes, or sliced bell peppers—snacks high in vitamin C. Better still, they look for locally grown fruits and vegetables at their target location. Particularly business travellers should be aware of their vitamin C demands, which can soar between stress, irregular meals and exposure to unfamiliar surroundings.

[Travel Hack: Stow some tangerines or oranges in your carry-on. They hydrate you and are like nature's travel insurance!

Though they are clever, our displays are causing some less-than-wise vitamin C problems. Every hour we spend gazing at phones, tablets, and laptops raises free radical generation in our bodies and eye strain. That blue glow everyone refers to? It might be raising our demand for antioxidants like vitamin C. Add to the stress of emails, alerts, and social media and our vitamin C supplies suffer greatly.

Actually, working from home has raised our vitamin C requirements as less outside time means less access to fresh food and sunlight. We seem to be living in a digital winter, and our bodies require extra help. The fix is here. Frequent screen breaks, lots of vitamin C-rich workplace snacks, and trying to consume fresh foods all throughout your digital day.

Your demand of vitamin C is largely influenced by your surroundings. City people generally require more as pollution raises oxidative stress on the body. Your body requires more antioxidant support, much as in a somewhat smokey area. With heating and cooling systems influencing vitamin C levels in our bodies, even indoor air can cause problems.

Furthermore influencing vitamin C in our diet is climate change. Although rising CO_2 levels could cause plants to grow larger, they sometimes lack nutrients. Vitamin C output of plants is affected by prolonged droughs, erratic rainfall, and high temperatures. Consider it as plants battling environmental stress to retain their vitamin content, same as humans do!

[Green Fact: Right on your windowsills, growing your own herbs or tiny veggies may supply fresh vitamin C].

For good reason, your brain is essentially the largest vitamin C hog in your body. Keeping the maximum concentration even in times of shortage, this vital organ stores around 15 times more vitamin C than other body components. Science indicates that vitamin C is vital in everything from mood control to memory development, from stress management to mental clarity; this preferred treatment is not random.

New studies have shown amazing links between brain performance and vitamin C levels. Exam season students and professionals working on demanding tasks typically display low vitamin C levels, which reflect what occurs under physical stress. Your brain seems to be running on vitamin C. Your brain needs more vitamin C the more psychologically stressful your day is.

[Brain Science: Vitamin C aids in the synthesis of neurotransmitters, the molecules enabling brain cells to interact. Insufficient vitamin C can cause this communication mechanism to slow down, therefore influencing mental function and mood.

Vitamin C's trip from farm to table is like a delicate ballet; one mistake and this valuable vitamin begins to vanish. The countdown starts the instant you chop an orange or fresh pepper. Diva of nutrients, vitamin C is vulnerable to light, heat, and air. Still, don't panic; with some clever cooking techniques, you may retain more of this essential vitamin in your dishes.

Storage really make a difference. The crisper drawer in your refrigerator is really a vitamin C preservation chamber, not simply a fancy division. Maintaining fruits and vegetables cold and somewhat damp allows them to keep their vitamin C content longer. Even the way you cut your produce counts: a sharp knife causes less damage to cells, therefore reducing the vitamin C loss.

[Kitchen Hack: Prepare your vitamin C-rich veggies immediately before eating; if you have to chop them ahead of time, refrigerate them in an airtight container. Including a splash of lemon juice helps stop vitamin loss.]

When your body heals, it starts to run like a vitamin C hungry machine. Your vitamin C demands soar whether your recovery from an accident, cold, or demanding exercise. Working extra to restore and heal damaged tissues, your body's construction staff is Your usual vitamin C intake may not be sufficient at these periods; you will need more resources for the rebuilding job.

Particularly athletes should be aware of their vitamin C levels. Intense training causes tiny muscle damage that requires repair; vitamin C is essential for this process of healing. Keeping a robust immune system is also rather important while your body is under physical stress. Even psychological tension raises your body's need for vitamin C; it's as if your cells are running a marathon even while you're still seated!

[Recovery Rule: During periods of recovery, your vitamin C demands may double or treble. Pay attention to the desires your body has for fresh veggies and citrus fruits; it knows what it needs!

Your body runs through vitamin C as a fire runs

through fuel when life becomes busy. Your adrenal glands burn vitamin C to generate stress hormones every time you're caught in traffic, juggling a deadline at work, or coping with any form of tension. This is why you could become ill following a particularly demanding period: your vitamin C supplies have been depleted just at the time your immune system most required them.

Constant emails, interminable meetings, social media overload, and 24/7 connectivity all raise our body's vitamin C needs, yet modern living seems to be meant to deplete this nutrient. Even "good" stress—that from workout or wedding planning—increases our demand. The answer is not only about grabbing pills but also about leading a lifestyle that routinely maintains and increases your vitamin C levels.

[Stress Fact: During trying circumstances, your body can burn up to two to three times more vitamin C. This is why many under stressed people yearn for oranges or other meals high in vitamin C!]

Vitamin C is not only another vitamin for sportsmen and fitness buffs; it's an indispensable component of their performance toolset. Your body generates extra free radicals—also known as cellular rust—during exercise; vitamin C helps balance these troublemakers. It's like having an internal housekeeper working extra during your exercise.

Here's where it becomes interesting, though: time

counts. Taking vitamin C shortly before a strenuous workout may actually offset some of the advantages of your activity. Instead, concentrate on taking enough vitamin C throughout your recovery phase, when your body is rebuilding and healing. Regular activity raises your general vitamin C requirements, hence athletes usually need more than those of inactive people.

[Athlete's Tip: Pack some vitamin C-rich snacks in your gym bag for post-workout recovery].

Living in our contemporary environment strains our stocks of vitamin C especially. Our demand for this protective vitamin is raised by environmental pollutants, UV light, and air pollution. Think of vitamin C as extra fortification against urban existence; city people often require more than their rural counterparts.

Vitamin C can even be depleted indoors. Our demand for and absorption of vitamin C may vary depending on artificial lighting, air conditioning, and warm air. Working in a high-rise structure or spending many hours indoors? Your needs for vitamin C might be more than you would believe. It's like having an additional protection against the unseen demands of contemporary life.

How can one find whether one is getting sufficient vitamin C? Your body provides faint messages. More often feeling weary? Recovering from exercises takes more time? Getting colds frequently? These might be hints that your vitamin C levels call for some work. Unlike extreme vitamin C insufficiency (scurvy), current deficiency is typically mild and stealthy.

The great thing about vitamin C is that your body tells clearly when you need more. Those sporadic appetites for strawberries or oranges are not entirely random; rather, your body is seeking a vitamin C boost. Consider it your internal dietitian delivering shopping lists based on desires.

[Body Signs: Your vitamin C requires care if your wounds heal slowly, bleeding gums or bruising easily.]

Various civilizations have interesting ways to receive their vitamin C. Fresh vegetables and citrus abound in Mediterranean diets. Asian cuisine sometimes calls for fruits and sprouts high in vitamin C. Typical Arctic diets deftly find vitamin C from uncommon sources like wild berries and seal liver.

Availability of vitamin C is being changed globally by climate change. Rising temperatures can lower the vitamin C concentration in plants; harsh weather can lower agricultural production. From growing more hardy crops to locating fresh vitamin C supplies, it is becoming a worldwide problem needing innovative answers.

[Cultural Note: Raw organ meats and kelp were the traditional sources of vitamin C for the Inuit, thereby demonstrating there is more than one approach to satisfy our needs].

Vitamin C is playing fascinating new functions according to scientists. Recent studies look at its possibilities in brain health, cancer therapy, and possibly aging prevention. Particularly pertinent in our current environment, several research imply vitamin C could help shield against radiation damage and consequences of air pollution.

Vitamin C research's future seems bright. We are continually learning fresh advantages of this vital nutrient from improved delivery technologies to knowledge of its function in genomic expression. With many more fascinating revelations coming, it feels as though we are still reading the beginning pages of vitamin C's narrative.

[Research Update: Scientists are investigating how vitamin C could shield against current environmental stresses like exposure to nanoparticles and 5G radiation.]

Although food should be your main supply of vitamin C, occasionally pills make sense. Not all supplements, meantime, are created equally. Timing counts and certain kinds are more absorbed than others. Generally speaking, morning dosages are better than evening ones; however, consuming vitamin C with meals increases absorption.

The secret is striking the proper balance for your

way of life. Beyond their diet, athletes, smokers, stressed executives, and pregnant women may need supplements. Remember though; more isn't always better. Your body only absorbs so much concurrently.

[Supplement Savvy: Search for supplements include bioflavonoids; they enable your body to better use vitamin C.]

Let's gather what we know about this amazing vitamin that does so much more than only ward against colds. One of the most adaptable health protectors found in nature, vitamin C is involved in many daily activities in your body. From bolstering your immune system like a devoted bodyguard to assisting in collagen building like a master builder, vitamin C shows itself to be quite helpful in ways our predecessors never would have anticipated.

Consider vitamin C as your body's master multi-tasker. Your immune system generates and activates white blood cells, your body's front-line defenses. Your skin needs collagen to keep you appearing young and aid in wound healing. Your brain keeps strong concentrations to support cognitive ability and emotional stability. It assists your heart to preserve the condition of blood vessels. In your muscles, it promotes recuperation and lessens oxidative damage brought on by activity. It's even involved in synthesis of several hormones and neurotransmitters, thereby acting as a vitamin's jack-of-all-traders.

Modern living presents special issues involving

vitamin C. From processed food to chronic stress, from air pollution to digital gadget radiation, our bodies deal with hitherto unheard-of pressures. These contemporary difficulties raise our vitamin C requirements just as our food sources may have less of this essential component because of environmental changes and current farming methods. Starting with less petrol in the tank, it's like sprinting a more difficult race.

The bright news is in some of the most mouthwatering meals on the planet, nature bundles vitamin C. This vitamin is most accessible in citrus fruits, berries, bell peppers, broccoli, and many other vibrantly colored vegetables and fruits. Though pills might be helpful when needed, your body accepts vitamin C from dietary sources more than from supplements. Recall those orange-related desires when battling a cold? That is the natural intelligence of your body working.

From its possible use in cancer treatment to its function in mental health, scientists are always finding fresh uses for vitamin C. Studies point to it supporting good aging and perhaps helping to shield against contemporary environmental stresses. Originally a basic remedy for scurvy, this vitamin has become among the most investigated and flexible one in current health research.

Features of Vitamin C include-

-Daily requirements change depending on lifestyle, degree of stress, and health state.

-Stress, pollution, smoke—even secondhand—also raise vitamin C needs.

-Usually speaking, food sources are better than supplements.

-Raw, fresh fruits and vegetables have the most vitamin C.

-Consistent, regular ingestion is preferable than sporadic high dosages.

Remember-

-Eat everyday a rainbow of fresh vegetables.

-Food storage and preparation help to reduce vitamin C loss.

-Pay attention to your body's cues to tell when you need more.

-Think about supplements during high-stress times.

-Pay particular attention during recovering from sickness.

Recall that vitamin C is about maximizing your health for modern life, not only about avoiding insufficiency. Whether your goals are professional stress management, athlete trying to improve recovery, or just someone trying to age healthily, knowing and maintaining your vitamin C needs is very essential for living in the modern world.

The value of vitamin C only increases as we meet fresh environmental and lifestyle issues. It is more important than ever as it supports basic physiological processes and helps against contemporary stresses. Not only are you avoiding scurvy by keeping appropriate vitamin C levels through food and judicious supplementation as needed, but you also are maximizing your body's capacity to meet the demands of modern life.

As sailors often took citrus fruits on lengthy trips, so too must we negotiate our current health path with vitamin C as a reliable friend. Vitamin C is still one of nature's most effective partners in our search for best health whether it's preventing seasonal diseases, helping mental clarity amid trying circumstances, or preserving skin health as we age.

Consider vitamin C as your body's devoted companion; constantly present when you need it, it works nonstop behind-the-scenes to keep you well. Understanding its several functions and making sure you have enough of it will help you not only support your health now but also invest in your wellbeing for

next years.

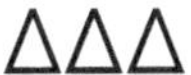

THE SUNSHINE VITAMIN-VITAMIN D

Imagine a vitamin so unique your body can make right now as sunlight touches your skin. Welcome to vitamin D, the only vitamin whose true nature is that of a hormone rather than merely a vitamin. While other vitamins have to be derived from food, your body is like a tiny vitamin D factory generating this essential component when sunlight comes into touch with your skin.

But contemporary life has disrupted this amazing natural system. More time spent inside, sunscreen use—which is essential for skin health—and urban living mean many of us lack adequate sun exposure to produce enough vitamin D. Low vitamin D levels are really considered to harm about a billion people worldwide. Think of it as a modern epidemic merely waiting for human awareness.

[Amazing Fact: 15 to 20 minutes of midday sun on your arms and legs will produce enough vitamin D for the day. But modern living often makes even this small amount challenging to get!]

Though its significance in bone health is well-known, that is merely the beginning. Recent research shows it influences everything from physical strength to cognitive function to immune system to mood regulation. Learning your reliable old flashlight is essentially like learning a complex Swiss Army knife!

Almost every cell in your body includes vitamin D receptors, suggesting that this chemical fulfills far more functions than once thought. Scientists are uncovering new, innovative ways that vitamin D influences human health from enhancing heart function to helping to prevent various cancers. This vitamin most of the times amazes us with its versatility.

[Research Note: Studies show vitamin D might cut the risk of everything from respiratory infections to autoimmune illnesses. Considering it's sometimes referred to be the "sunshine vitamin," many sectors of life gain from a glimmer of hope.]

Our global vitamin D problem transcends beyond spending too much time inside. To get the same amount of vitamin D as fairer complexion, dark skin need more sun exposure. Those residing in northern latitudes may not get enough UVB rays for the production of vitamin D even if they spend time outside. Add to air pollution filtering sunlight to obtain the perfect storm for vitamin D insufficiency.

Working from home has complicated things. Maybe your early trip or midday walk was providing more vitamin D than you would have guessed. Many of us now walk from bed to a workstation or sofa, without seeing sunshine. We appear to be all living in an indoor winter all the time.

[Urban Fact: Tall buildings block sunlight and more time spent indoors indicates that city dwellers are more prone to be vitamin D deficient.]

The way your body generates vitamin D is quite astonishingly sophisticated. UVB rays hit your skin and start a series of events turning cholesterol into vitamin D3. This then goes to your liver, where it becomes more palable. Your kidneys finally convert it into the super-powered form your body can use.

The problem is, however, this operation is less

effective than it used to be. Your body generates vitamin D based on age, weight, skin color, even the time of day. It's like running a factory whereby extremely specific conditions determine whether excellent functioning is possible.

Your body can generate 10,000–25,000 IU of vitamin D in just 15 minutes of total-body sun exposure!

Ever noticed that bright days make your mood better? That is not simply psychological; management of mood depends on vitamin D, which is absolutely essential. Studies of seasonal affective disorder (SAD) substantially correlate with vitamin D levels. Those winter blues might be your body yearning for more vitamin D.

Your brain is full of vitamin D receptors in areas linked to anxiety and depression. Declining vitamin D levels might affect your serotonin levels, the "happy hormone." Think of vitamin D as the sunlight boost your brain needs to keep your mood brilliant even in non-weather situations.

[Mood Fact: Studies show sad people typically have low vitamin D levels; in certain cases, supplementation might help to improve mood.]

Like the general of your immune system, vitamin D maintains discipline and directs soldiers. When your immune cells are needed, they become more active; when they are overreacting, they become calmer.

This dual purpose makes prevention of autoimmune illnesses as well as fight of infections absolutely important.

During cold and flu season, maybe as important as hand washing is vitamin D levels. Studies have linked reduced risks of respiratory infections to higher vitamin D levels. It is like having extra defense against seasonal infections.

Let's not undervalue vitamin D's great relevance for skeletal health even if it does considerably more than merely build bones. You can eat all the foods heavy in calcium in the world without vitamin D and yet have weak bones. This is so because vitamin D guides calcium into your bones where it is needed like a security guard.

This gets much more important as we become older. After thirty we start to naturally lose bone mass; without enough vitamin D this process accelerates. If post-menopausal women wish to maintain their bone strength, they especially need to know their vitamin D level.

[Bone Fact: Vitamin D works with calcium to reduce the incidence of osteoporosis; nonetheless, it depends on enough magnesium to function since it is a three-way interaction for bone health.]

In terms of physical performance, vitamin D is almost your body's secret weapon. Ideal vitamin D levels generally translate into faster, stronger, more efficient athletes than their peers who are deficient. This extends beyond professional athletes; even everyday gym-goers and weekend warriors benefit from proper dosages of vitamin D. Your muscles have vitamin D receptors; consequently, when these receptors are deficient of sunshine vitamin, strength and performance may decrease.

Studies show that vitamin D is very important for both growth and strength of muscle fibers. Low levels might result in higher risk of injury, muscle weakness, and slower healing periods. For senior people specifically, maintaining enough vitamin D becomes extremely crucial as it maintains muscular power and coordination, therefore reducing falls. Professional sports teams nowadays frequently monitor the vitamin D levels of their athletes, especially in the winter when sun exposure is limited.

Consider vitamin D as your muscles' maintenance coordinator. It assists damage repair following activities; it also stimulates protein synthesis for muscle growth and even helps reduce inflammation. If your vitamin D levels are low, post-workout pain might be really extreme. Many athletes find faster recovery times and better endurance by optimizing their vitamin D levels.

Research in sports science show that athletes with optimal vitamin D levels have up to 10-20% faster response times and improved muscular power output!

Research has recently discovered amazing connections between vitamin D levels and cardiovascular health. Low vitamin D has been linked to high blood pressure, heart disease, and other cardiovascular diseases as well as to other It's like having a wall around your heart; that shield disappears when vitamin D levels drop.

Vitamin D helps to control blood pressure by means of hormone regulation. It also helps maintain the integrity of blood vessels and reduces inflammation all over the cardiovascular system. Ironically, some research suggest that vitamin D can help stop the buildup of calcium in arteries given its role in helping calcium create bones!

Beyond the heart itself, vitamin D helps regulate cholesterol levels and encourages proper blood sugar metabolism. It is quite clear that this solar vitamin is really essential for keeping your cardiovascular system in optimal operation. Even your blood vessels reveal the need of vitamin D for circulation by having receptors of this vitamin.

[Heart Health Note: Maintaining optimal vitamin D levels may be as important for heart health as regular exercise and a nutritious diet!]

Your brain loves oxygen roughly equally to vitamin D! Important areas of the brain, including those connected to memory, learning, and emotional processing, contain lots of vitamin D receptors according recent studies. It's like having a sunshine switch in your brain controlling mood as well as all other element of cognitive capacity.

Scientists have found interesting links between vitamin D and lifelong brain performance. Correct brain development of the fetus during pregnancy depends on enough vitamin D, which is extremely necessary. Early on it promotes learning and cognitive development. Keeping proper vitamin D levels helps people avoid age-related cognitive decline and maybe reduce their risk of various neurological diseases.

One rather amazing connection occurs between mental health and vitamin D. Higher risk of depression, anxiety, and seasonal affective disorder

(SAD) has been linked to low levels. According to certain research, the present epidemic of mental health issues may have some influence on a general vitamin D deficiency. Think of vitamin D as the emotional support food for your brain; low levels might lead to mental frailty.

[Brain Science: Vitamin D helps protect neurons; it also increases the creation of several essential neurotransmitters, including those controlling mood and cognitive abilities.]

Let's talk about what happens when your body runs low on vitamin D; this is more often than you would know. Vitamin D deficiency might be mild unlike other vitamin shortages that show obvious symptoms quickly. Usually it presents as vague symptoms like weariness, muscle weakness, or recurrent infections. Many people attribute their symptoms to stress or busy schedules without realizing they are low in this essential vitamin.

The real concern is from the long-term effects of vitamin D deficiency. From steady low levels, bone problems, higher risk of autoimmune illnesses, more vulnerability to infections, and even quicker aging can all follow. Children with vitamin D deficiency can develop rickets, a condition whereby their bones become mushy and twisted. In adults, it can cause osteoporosis, muscle weakness, and increased fall risk.

Modern living's elements contribute to the commonness of insufficiency in recent times. Sunscreen lowers the production of vitamin D even if it helps prevent skin cancer. Your risk of deficiency inside, in northern latitudes, increases with darker skin, fat, and age. It's like a perfect storm of components weakening your body's vitamin D synthesis.

[Muscle weakness, bone pain, frequent infections, weariness, and mood changes might all point to low vitamin D levels.]

Beyond only getting a blood test, knowing your vitamin D level enables you to know what those levels mean and how best to maximize them. The usual test measures 25-hydroxyvitamin D levels; most experts agree that readings below 20 ng/mL suggest insufficiency; the sweet spot for health benefits is between 30-50 ng/mL even although there is much debate on optimal levels.

Correcting your levels requires more than just lounging in the sun or ingesting medicines. It is about finding the right balance for your specific needs. Factors like skin color, age, weight, latitude, season, and overall health affect your need of vitamin D. While some people might need additional vitamins, others can maintain healthy levels by diet just and sun exposure.

Furthermore important is time of vitamin D

consumption. Since it's fat-soluble, it improves absorption when taken with meals heavy in fat. Morning pills could be more helpful than evening ones as they mirror the usual schedule of sun exposure. Regular testing allows you to hone your plan and ensures that you are maintaining appropriate levels all year round.

[Testing Tip: The best time to check vitamin D levels is toward the end of winter, when they typically are lowest; this offers a "worst-case scenario" baseline.]

Let's talk about how one organically receives vitamin D: from sunlight. But this is more complex than just leaving the house. Timing is quite important. Typically, when UVB levels are highest, the sweet spot for vitamin D synthesis occurs between 10 AM and 3 PM. This is where it gets interesting, though: more often shorter periods of sun exposure might be better than sporadic longer sessions.

Also really crucial is your skin type. Darker skin calls for more sun than white skin if one wants the same degree of vitamin D. Another factor is age; with the same daily exposure, elder skin produces less vitamin D. Location also contributes; living above 37 degrees latitude (maybe Boston or Rome) produces UVB levels inadequate for winter vitamin D production.

Real too is the conundrum about clothing. Sunscreen lowers the production of vitamin D even if it is vitally necessary in preventing skin cancer. The fix is right here. Several experts suggest spending several minutes in the sun before applying sunscreen. Think of it as a quick change for your body's vitamin D factory before putting on the safety gear.

[Sun Smart: Exposing your arms for 10 to 15 minutes and rolling up your sleeves during lunch break might provide more vitamin D than a glass of fortified milk!]

Mostly found in eggs yolks, fatty fish, and certain mushrooms, nature lacks many natural dietary sources of vitamin D. For this reason, several countries fortify meals such milk, cereal, and orange juice. Nature seemed to provide us few dietary backup options and meant for us to get most of our vitamin D from the Sun.

Among the pack in vitamin D content are fatty fish. A meal of wild-caught salmon will supply more vitamin D than most people get in a day. The vitamin D in the egg yolks of chicken reared outdoors exceeded those of hens raised indoors. Under UV exposure, certain mushrooms may produce substantial amounts of vitamin D; they are like little vitamin D factories!

Fascinatingly, the vitamin D in animal meals (D3) is more strong than in diets based on plants (D2). This especially challenges vegans and vegetarians, who could need more on supplements or fortified foods. Now some innovative companies are producing vegan D3 from lichen, providing a plant-based replacement.

[Food Fact: Wild-caught salmon can have up to four times more vitamin D than farmed salmon – it's like getting a sunny extra in your seafood!]

About vitamin D tablets, not every one of them is manufactured equally. The form counts; typically, D3, cholecalciferol is more effective than D2, erocalciferol. Although the RDA might be 600–800 IU daily, some experts suggest that higher doses may be needed for optimal health, especially for those who run insufficiency risk.

Crucially also are timing and combination. Since vitamin D is fat-soluble, taking it with meals heavy in fat helps absorption. Some studies suggest that morning vitamin D consumption could more fairly represent patterns of natural sun exposure. Moreover crucial is the magnesium relationship as without adequate magnesium vitamin D cannot perform as it should.

Quality control in supplements varies widely. Look for goods from reputable manufacturers who have had third-party evaluations. Some supplements combine vitamin D with complementing minerals like vitamin K2 to help ensure that calcium accumulates in bones rather than arteries.

[Supplement Savvy: Look for supplements containing D3 with K2; they work for cardiovascular and bone health like a great team].

Some groups should give their vitamin D situation

particular thought. Not only for themselves but also for the bone health and cognitive development of their growing child, pregnant women need more vitamin D. Older persons usually spend less time outside, their skin generates less vitamin D, and their systems do not properly metabolize vitamin D. These provide a triple hurdle.

Sometimes up to six times longer than individuals with lighter complexion, people with darker skin require far more sun exposure to generate sufficient vitamin D. Another problem is obesity as less vitamin D is accessible for the body to consume since it accumulates in fat tissue. To maintain their higher physical needs, even athletes—who spend time outside—may require extra vitamin D.

Workers on night shifts deal more difficultly with vitamin D. Their inverted calendar causes them to miss the hours of maximum sunshine; artificial light does not boost vitamin D synthesis. It's like living in constant winter and calls for meticulous supplements plans.

[Population Note: Studies reveal that up to 80% of senior residents in nursing homes might be vitamin D deficient, so this is a major health issue.]

Your vitamin D demands vary with the seasons and call for varied approaches all year long. While modest sun exposure could be sufficient in summer, winter calls for a more aggressive strategy. Consider it like getting your automobile ready for various driving environments; different seasons call for different approaches.

Fall is the time to stockpile your vitamin D before winter arrives. This might require raising supplement dosages or spending more time outside under strong enough sun. Winter calls most supplements, particularly in northern latitudes when UVB rays are rare.

Spring presents unique difficulties; many people have lowest vitamin D levels following winter. Your body requires time to replenish its vitamin D supplies, just as one would emerge from hibernation. Though balance is important to prevent sun damage, summer presents the best chance for natural vitamin D synthesis.

[Seasonal Tip: To better understand your body's seasonal rhythms, think about having your vitamin D levels checked at the end of winter and end of summer.]

Fascinating connections between vitamin D levels and certain disorders have lately been found by study. Reduced vitamin D levels are linked to higher risk of autoimmune diseases, certain malignancies, heart disease, and respiratory infections. It is like having a master key influencing several locks in the health system of your body.

Particularly fascinating is the immunological link as vitamin D controls adaptive and natural immunity. It can strengthen your immune system's capacity to fight off infections and help avoid overreaction—as in autoimmune diseases—of your immune system. This double function makes general immunological balance absolutely vital.

New studies point to vitamin D possibly helping to prevent or control ailments like Type 2 diabetes, multiple sclerosis, and even some mental illnesses. New findings on how this solar vitamin affects human health abound every year.

[Research Update: Studies suggest that ideal vitamin D levels may cut some cancer risk by up to 50%!]

Vitamin D and exercise have an amazing association. Outdoor physical activity has two advantages: you get the exercise and sun exposure-related vitamin D. But this narrative has much to tell. Enough vitamin D can enhance exercise performance; exercise may help your body more effectively use vitamin D.

Athletes should give their vitamin D situation more thought. Low levels have effects on bone health, recuperation time, and muscular strength. When their vitamin D levels are ideal, even leisurely exercisers may find better performance. Consider vitamin D as part of your training diet; it is just as vital for muscular health as protein.

Exercise indoors vs. outside raises various vitamin D

issues. Although a gym session would be excellent for fitness, including some outdoor training sessions helps preserve naturally occurring vitamin D levels. Winter athletes have particular difficulties and usually need extra supplements to keep ideal levels.

[Exercise Fact: Studies reveal that athletes' muscular strength may increase with vitamin D supplements, therefore lowering their injury risk.]

For vitamin D levels, our current way of life presents special difficulties. Blue light from screens can throw off our circadian cycles, which can influence our bodies' vitamin D metabolism. UVB rays can be blocked by air pollution, therefore compromising our capacity to generate vitamin D even outside.

Working from home has shifted our solar exposure schedule. Less inadvertent sun exposure results from everyday travels lost outdoors lunch breaks. Considering natural light exposure is now part of smart workplace design as it is so important for vitamin D and general wellness.

The answer is not to give up contemporary amenities but rather to modify our vitamin D plans for current living. This might entail planning brief outside breaks during peak sun, using light treatment in the winter, or changing supplement schedules depending on way of life.

[Modern Life Tip: Consider it as your vitamin D coffee break: schedule a daily alarm for a 10-15 minute outdoor break during peak sunshine hours].

Let's look at how vitamin D aids detoxification and cellular health. Appropriate vitamin D levels support the normal operation of your body's detox processes. Think of vitamin D as your body's housekeeper, cleaning cells and maintaining normal cell turnover. Research show it may even help protect against daily environmental toxins.

Vitamin D helps control liver activity of detoxification-related enzymes. This is really important considering our interaction to various pollutants, chemicals, and processed meals. Your skin, being the largest detox organ, benefits from ample vitamin D as well to maintain its barrier function and repair mechanisms.

[Detox Detail: Perfect vitamin D levels will help up to 30% of your body's natural detoxification systems to be enhanced, therefore enhancing cellular cleaning and renewal.]

Unbelievably, vitamin D regulates circadian rhythm and sleep quality. New research show brain vitamin D receptors controlling our sleep-wake cycles. Those with adequate vitamin D levels often report better quality and more consistent sleeping habits.

The timing of your vitamin D intake—that from pills or sunlight—may affect your internal clock. Apart from vitamin D, early sun exposure helps to set daily circadian rhythm. This is the reason exposure to morning light generally produces better nighttime sleep.

Lack of sleep might affect the way your body absorbs vitamin D, therefore creating a dangerous cycle of shortage. Breaking this cycle might require observation of vitamin D levels as well as sleep habits.

[Sleep Science: Morning sun exposure can enhance nocturnal sleep quality by up to 40% by means of its effect on both vitamin D production and circadian rhythms].

While most of us link vitamin D to sun exposure, it really has numerous functions in the health of skin.

Found in your skin cells, vitamin D receptors help regulate immune system response, cell growth, and healing. For conditions ranging from aging to acne, vitamin D is therefore critically essential.

Vitamin D helps regulate skin inflammation, thereby possibly treating conditions including psoriasis and eczema. It also helps the skin's antibacterial defense system, therefore preventing infections. Particularly interesting are the anti-aging properties as vitamin D protects DNA repair processes in skin cells.

Many doctors now counsel balanced sun exposure for optimum skin condition, challenging the "avoid sun at all costs" approach. The trick is to get the right balance between protecting from UV damage and getting enough vitamin D.

[Skin Science: Vitamin D boosts skin repair genes capable of up to 25% decrease in visible age signs].

The link between brain-vitamin D goes beyond basic mood. Vitamin D receptors abound all across the brain, particularly in areas linked to memory and learning. Studies show that vitamin D supports overall brain function and could even assist against age-related cognitive decline.

For professionals as well as students, especially at times of intense mental activity, maintaining optimum vitamin D levels might aid. The vitamin helps to manufacture neurotransmitters and maintains the state of brain cells. Some studies even show a link between vitamin D status and cognitive ability.

As we become older, maintaining enough vitamin D becomes increasingly more crucial for brain function. Perhaps reducing the prevalence of neurodegenerative illnesses, the vitamin protects the brain from oxidative stress and inflammation.

[Studies show that optimal vitamin D levels might boost cognitive performance by up to 20% in specific activities.]

There is fascinating and varied connection between vitamin D and gut health. Although vitamin D promotes the growth of beneficial bacteria and supports the preservation of a healthy gut barrier, your gut flora can influence the way effectively you absorb and use vitamin D.

Along with helping to manage inflammation in the stomach, vitamin D strengthens the immune system there. This is quite important as over seventy percent of your immune system resides in your gut. People who have digestive issues usually have low vitamin D levels, which might cause a probable cycle necessitating both directions of treatment.

New research highlight how vitamin D improves gut health, so affecting the gut-brain axis and hence impacting all aspect of life, including immune system. Some probiotics even help to improve vitamin D absorption and utilization.

[Gut Health Note: By maximising vitamin D levels, gut barrier function can be up to 60% increased, therefore supporting better nutrient absorption and immunological function.]

Let's see how vitamin D directs your hormonal symphony. Being a hormone by itself, vitamin D interacts practically every hormonal system in your body. It controls thyroid function, preserves appropriate insulin production, and influences reproductive hormones. Think of it as the conductor keeping each of your hormonal players in tune.

Particularly women's hormonal health benefits from

optimal vitamin D. It can help manage monthly cycles, increase fertility, and ease menopausal changes. From brain development to bone growth, enough vitamin D becomes rather important for both mother and growing fetus during pregnancy.

Vitamin D affects testosterone production and reproductive health in men as well. Low vitamin D levels have been linked to lowered testosterone and fertility as well. Older men and sportsmen should concentrate primarily on their vitamin D level in order to optimize hormones.

[Hormone Fact: Particularly with regard to thyroid and reproductive hormones, appropriate vitamin D levels can help to enhance up to 40% of hormonal balance.]

Children's needs for vitamin D call especially for special consideration. During growth spurts, vitamin D demands increase to support optimal immune system development and bone building. While selective eating may limit dietary sources, modern indoor life makes it difficult for youngsters to get enough sunshine.

Level of vitamin D might also affect performance in the classroom. Studies show that children with adequate vitamin D levels often score better academically and have less behavioral issues. The vitamin's role in brain development and function becomes increasingly important throughout critical learning years.

The combination of physical activity and vitamin D helps children grow. Outdoor play gives both sun exposure and exercise, therefore promoting excellent growth. Children's vitamin D level regulation has gotten more challenging in part from greater screen time and indoor living.

[Child Development Note: Children with optimal vitamin D levels show up to 30% better on cognitive development.]

Athletes present a special case when it comes to vitamin D needs. While maybe lowering sun exposure, indoor exercise increases vitamin

D requirements. Ideal vitamin D levels allow performance indicators including response speed, muscle strength, and recovery all to go well.

Athletes in endurance sports particularly find challenges. Early morning or evening when UVB levels are low might be extensive training hours. Though convenient, indoor training facilities stop natural vitamin D production. Maintaining performance levels rely on extremely necessary strategic supplements.

Enough vitamin D benefits recovery as well as in injury prevention. The interaction of the vitamin with muscle performance, bone health, and inflammatory regulation determines athletic lifespan most importantly. While planning their workout, even recreational athletes should consider their vitamin D status.

[Studies show up to 15% boost in measures of athletic performance at optimal vitamin D levels.]

As we age, our vitamin D needs change; our ability to produce and use it also decreases. While absorption and conversion in the body may decline, skin loses effectiveness in producing vitamin D from sunlight. Still, the need for vitamin D definitely increases with aging.

Bone health becomes increasingly important as one ages, and the role of vitamin D in calcium absorption and bone metabolism is even more vital. Enough vitamin D helps maintain bone density and reduce fall risk in combination with weight-bearing exercise.

Furthermore very dependent on vitamin D are cognitive functions and emotional stability in aging. The neuroprotective qualities of the vitamin and its role in the production of neurotransmitters become extremely important as we age in maintaining mental clarity and emotional balance.

[Aging Insight: Maintaining adequate vitamin D levels can up to 25% aid to fight against age-related decline in several functions].

Environmental factors and climate change seem to

be surprisingly influencing our vitamin D level: Rising air pollution filters UVB radiation, therefore reducing the natural production of vitamin D even in outdoor settings. Our possibilities for solar exposure and outdoor activities rely on variations in the temperature.

One has particular challenges living in an urban location. Tall buildings create "vitamin D shadows," therefore lowering solar exposure even during outside activities. The solution requires for creative approaches of sun protection and complementing strategies. Currently under discussion in numerous locations are "vitamin D zones" for urban planning.

Furthermore changing our vitamin D level is indoor air quality and lighting. While current LED lighting is energy-efficient, its benefits are fewer than those of natural sunlight. Some progressive companies are designing "vitamin D-friendly" indoor lighting solutions.

[Environmental Note: Urban pollution can reduce sunlight's vitamin D producing ability by up to 60%.]

Investigating further the complex connection between vitamin D and stress is definitely worth it. Low vitamin D levels might, meantime, make you more sensitive to the negative effects of stress, therefore creating a challenging cycle.

Vitamin D receptors abound in your adrenal glands, which produce stress hormone. Appropriate levels of vitamin D help these glands to function as they should, therefore reducing your stress sensitivity. From employment pressures to marital issues to other life obligations, your vitamin D needs might climb significantly during times of extreme stress.

Not only is mental stress significant; physical stress from illness, surgery, or intense exercise can also increase vitamin D requirements. Think of vitamin D as your body's stress reliever; your need for resilience rises with rising stress level.

Studies show that ongoing stress can drain vitamin D supplies up to 50% faster than normal!

Let's examine attentively the contribution vitamin D

makes to immune system operation. Your immune system's cells include vitamin D receptors, which helps this vitamin help coordinate immunological reactions. Like a competent conductor leading an orchestra, vitamin D ensures your immune system responds properly to challenges without overreacting.

Your body creates natural antibiotics to combat infections; vitamin D helps to make antimicrobial peptides in some degree. It also regulates inflammatory responses, thereby maybe reducing the risk of autoimmune illnesses. Seasonal changes in immunity often coincide with fluctuations in vitamin D levels all year long.

The connection between vitamin D and respiratory health especially is fascinating. Since vitamin D levels normally drop in winter, more upper respiratory infections follow. This is not a fortuitous event; the health of respiratory tract linings depends critically on vitamin D.

[Immune Insight: Ideal vitamin D levels can provide up to 40% improvement in immune function efficacy.]

Body weight and vitamin D have a somewhat complex connection. Since vitamin D may be retained in adipose tissue, the body finds it less easily available. Higher body fat people might thus need more vitamin D to maintain appropriate blood levels.

When vitamin D levels are optimal, attempts at weight loss might be more successful. The vitamin helps with metabolism and may regulate appetite. Some studies suggest that correcting a vitamin D deficit might enable more long-lasting and simple weight loss.

The cycle may go both ways: losing weight lets your body access more vitamin D. On a limited diet, rapid weight loss might, however, temporally increase vitamin D requirements as the body adjusts.

Higher body fat people may need up to two to three times more vitamin D to attain appropriate blood levels [Note on weight control].

Unique vitamin D problems exist for many populations all throughout the world. Those who live near the equator might cope with extra difficulties such indoor living or cultural clothing choices even if they have enough of sun exposure. Northern residents may have diets heavy in foods strong in vitamin D, such as fatty fish but limited sun exposure.

From sun exposure patterns to fish liver consumption, indigenous civilizations often have basic ways of ensuring enough vitamin D. Modern living has disturbed many of these established patterns and creates new challenges for maintaining optimal vitamin D levels.

Changing with climate is global vitamin D status. Variations in temperature, greater air pollution, and altering lifestyle choices all influence our ability to maintain adequate vitamin D levels. Some countries are responding with national programs on vitamin D fortification.

[Global Fact: Vitamin D inadequacy affects over a billion people worldwide, thereby posing a significant worldwide health concern.]

Regarding vitamin D, interesting advances are under place. New supplement delivery systems seem to offer better absorption. Smart devices that detect UV exposure and project vitamin D production are now on sale. Some companies are developing indoor lighting systems with vitamin D content boosted.

Different people absorb vitamin D depending on their genetic makeup. This knowledge is producing more tailored suggestions regarding supplements. Some research are investigating vitamin D analogues, modified forms of the vitamin with putative medical value.

The future could provide foods high in vitamin D thanks to biofortification, UV-treated mushrooms becoming more common, even "vitamin D windows" permitting beneficial UVB rays but limiting harmful radiation.

[Tech Note: New vitamin D measuring technologies

can presently track your own production with up to 95% accuracy.]

Vitamin D demands vary greatly across life, much as chapters in a book. Strong bones and a strong immune system development depend on vitamin D all through infancy. Teenagers' years demand for additional vitamin D to support rapid increase of bone density. Young people need it to maintain reproductive health and preserve optimum bone mass.

Pregnancy presents a different vitamin D story: needs surge as the developing infant depends on this vitamin for everything from brain development to bone growth. For optimum health, mother and child both need suitable levels following childbirth. Middle age brings distinct challenges as the body's need for muscle and bone support increases while natural production falls.

Senior years need even more careful attention to vitamin D levels. The skin's ability to produce vitamin D may decrease by up to 75% compared to younger years. Combining this with less outdoor time and reduced absorption efficiency creates a perfect storm for scarcity.

There are especially difficulties for vitamin D in city living. Tall buildings create urban canyons that reduce sun exposure, air pollution filters UVB rays, and indoor lifestyles further diminish vitamin D synthesis. Living in perpetual darkness begs for creative ideas to maintain proper levels.

Starting with vitamin D considerations is wise urban design. Aimed to improve safe sun exposure; various cities are creating "sun spaces" in public parks and squares. Office buildings have alfresco sections and vitamin D-friendly lighting systems. Even urban gardening is involved; UV-exposed mushrooms are starting to become a hot source of vitamin D.

For city dwellers, the solution often consists of judicious sun exposure during lunch breaks, well selected supplements, and knowledge of foods heavy in vitamin D. To enable city inhabitants optimize their sun exposure, some forward-looking companies are even developing "urban vitamin D tracking apps".

[Urban Fact: City dwellers might have up to 40% less vitamin D than their national counterparts.]

More complex interplay exists between vitamin D and sleep than initially thought. New research indicates that vitamin D receptors abound in areas of the brain in charge of regulating sleep. Low vitamin D levels have been associated with both daytime tiredness and insomnia. It's like a broken dimmer switch in the everyday rhythm of your body.

Recovering from an accident, a disease, or an exercise also depends in part on vitamin D level. During recovery, the vitamin maintains muscle activity, reduces inflammation, and promotes tissue mending. Athletes are finding that optimal vitamin D levels can reduce injury risk and speed recovery periods.

Enough vitamin D promotes even emotional recovery. Recovering from emotional challenges depends on the vitamin as it helps modulate mood and stress response. Think of it as your body's healing sidekick working behind the scenes to help with bounce-back.

[Sleep Science: Perfect vitamin D levels can lead to up to 35% greater sleep quality.]

Vitamin D cannot operate alone; it is part of a complex network of nutrients that supports one another. Magnesium determines how vitamin D is metabolised; without enough of it, vitamin D cannot operate as it should. Working with vitamin D, vitamin K2 guarantees that calcium ends up in bones rather than arteries. Zinc helps the body to activate its vitamin D.

Working together, the fat-soluble vitamins (A, D, E, and K) complement one another in terms of functions and help to maintain the body in balance. This is why getting nutrients from complete meals typically works better than isolated tablets; you get the whole bundle of supporting nutrients.

Also involved in vitamin D function are your gut bacteria. A good flora helps absorption and usage of vitamin D. Probiotics, fermented foods, and gut health support can assist to enhance your vitamin D level.

[Synergy Note: Up to 60% improvement in vitamin D effectiveness can come from combined nutrition programs].

New discoveries broadening the area of vitamin D Researchers are uncovering novel roles for this vitamin in everything, from athletic performance to brain activity. Gene studies are helping to clarify why some people respond differently to vitamin D supplementation. Some studies examine how vitamin D could affect longevity and good aging.

New delivery methods are in researched from more absorbable vitamins to foods boosted in vitamin D. Some academics are working on personalized dosing algorithms that include individual factors like health condition, lifestyle, and heredity. Standard in the future might be vitamin D monitoring gadgets, as widespread as fitness monitors.

From autoimmune diseases to mental health problems, clinical research on vitamin D's therapeutic potential in various conditions is under progress. The results might change our view of this nutrient's overall health and disease preventive role.

[Research Update: Under examination fresh applications of vitamin D in human health by about 4,000 researchers worldwide.]

Since vitamin D is your body's defense system, let's look at how it guards against various diseases. Recent research show it may help prevent colon, breast, and prostate malignancies among other types of cancer. Because it may regulate cell growth and death (apoptosis), the vitamin is a powerful agent in cancer prevention.

Beyond cancer, vitamin D has promise in either preventing or managing autoimmune disorders. Multiple sclerosis, rheumatoid arthritis, type 1 diabetes, and vitamin D level all show links. It's like having an internal peacekeeper supporting your immune system not attacking itself.

Studies suggest optimum vitamin D levels might reduce autoimmune disease risk by up to 40% and certain cancer risk by up to 50%.

Our ever more digital style of life has surprisingly effects on vitamin D level. The circadian cycles that screen blue light throws off affect vitamin D absorption in our bodies. Working remotely has reduced our unintentional sun exposure; those brief walks to lunch or commutes used to create some vitamin D production have less effect.

Smart homes and companies are including more and more circadian lighting systems that strive to emulate natural light cycles. To encourage outdoor time during higher UV levels, several creative companies are adding "vitamin D breaks" into their workplace wellness campaigns.

The rise of e-sports and gaming culture raises significant issues because many young people spend formerly unheard-of amounts of time indoors. This shift demands new strategies to maintain vitamin D levels in our increasingly more virtual world.

Climate change is changing our vitamin D narrative in complex ways. Rising temperatures might push people to spend more time indoors, even while increasing air pollution can block UVB rays even during outside time. Changing weather patterns affect traditional seasonal events that formerly naturally generated vitamin D.

In certain places longer winters or more cloud cover are reducing natural vitamin D production opportunities. Some areas find too much heat makes midday sun exposure impossible. These changes demand for us to adjust our vitamin D intake based on the environment.

Scientists are looking at how climate change may affect dietary sources of vitamin D from changes in fish migratory patterns to impacts on mushroom formation. Knowing these changes will help us to be prepared for forthcoming vitamin D requirements.

Your DNA remarkably affects the vitamin D processing of your body. While some people take vitamin D more slowly, others are genetically "fast metabolizers," quick absorbing and using it. Understanding your genetic type can allow you to explain why you need either more or less vitamin D than others.

Individual differences abound in VDR (Vitamin

D Receptor) genes. These variations affect how efficiently your body absorbs vitamin D independent of blood level. Some people may need higher dosages to get the same benefits depending on their genetic makeup.

[Genetic Note: Up to 30% of people have genetic variations affecting their vitamin D processing, which calls for customized supplement programs.]

Among the key inflammatory regulators in your body is vitamin D. Think of it as a firefighter trying to extinguish inflammatory "fires" all throughout your body. Common in modern life, persistent inflammation can increase vitamin D needs and simultaneously impair your body's usage of this mineral.

Stress, a poor diet, or environmental toxins can all cause low-grade inflammation that sets off a vicious cycle resulting in a vitamin D deficiency. Often stopping this cycle requires simultaneous control of vitamin D level and inflammation.

Recent research suggest that vitamin D might be able to regulate inflammatory illnesses ranging from inflammatory bowel disease to arthritis. Nowadays, treating chronic inflammatory illnesses mostly depends on this.

Regarding vitamin D, top sportsmen should exercise especially carefulness. Early morning or evening exercise sessions, indoor training facilities, and protective clothing can all serve to limit natural vitamin D generation; performance expectations, recovery needs, and training intensity can also all help to boost vitamin D needs.

Clearly, optimal vitamin D levels enhance response times, physical strength, and endurance among performance criteria. In an optimal state of vitamin D, recovery from intense exercise sessions might be faster. Levels of vitamin D may influence even mental focus and competitive edge.

[Athlete Edge: Ideal vitamin D levels help elite athletes show up to 30% better recovery rates and reduced injury risk.]

Children's vitamin D demands vary substantially during times of development. Rapid bone building, immune system maturation, and cognitive development all depend on appropriate vitamin D. Modern indoor life and screen use make meeting these needs challenging.

School performance shows interesting correlation with vitamin D level. Not just conduct but also attention, learning ability may change depending on vitamin D levels. These days, several universities have "sunshine breaks" scheduled everyday.

Childhood obesity presents special challenges for vitamin D status as additional body fat can trap this fat-soluble vitamin and limit its availability for use.

Pregnancy creates strange vitamin D demands. For the developing child, appropriate bone growth, brain development, and immune system programming all depend on this vitamin. Maternal vitamin D level during pregnancy can influence birth weight as well as subsequent health results.

From conception to age 2, the first 1000 days of life provide a critical window for vitamin D. Appropriate levels during this period might help programs provide long-term benefits for health. Mother and kid both have great need for attentive attention to vitamin D levels during this essential era.

[Pregnancy Priority: Perfect vitamin D levels during pregnancy might decrease problems by up to 25%.]

Aging brings a number of issues regarding vitamin D. While absorption and conversion in the body may decrease, skin loses ability to synthesize vitamin D. But the requirement for vitamin D actually increases with age for cognitive function, muscle strength, and bone health.

Since vitamin D is necessary for maintaining muscle strength and balance, fall prevention becomes a key concern for senior citizens. Enough vitamin D along with appropriate exercise will assist to drastically reduce fall risk.

Perfect vitamin D levels also aid with memory and

cognitive capacity in aging, so this vitamin is crucial for strategies of healthy aging.

Recent international events have underscored the significance of maintaining optimal vitamin D level throughout crises. Vitamin D levels in crises can be influenced by stress, minimal food choices, and prolonged inside time.

One should consider vitamin D sources some attention during emergency preparedness. Important elements of emergency planning become shelf-stable vitamin D-rich meals, supplement supplies, and safe sun exposure practices.

Today's environmental toxins can interfere with vitamin D's activity. Some chemicals, particularly endocrine disruptors, may interfere with the way vitamin D receptors function or metabolism is handled. Apart from UVB protection, air pollution could increase the need for vitamin D by the body.

Plastics, pesticides, and industrial toxins might interact complexly with vitamin D pathways. Knowing these links becomes crucial for appropriate vitamin D level in the modern environment.

Some environmental contaminants can reduce the vitamin D efficacy by up to 40%, even in circumstances where blood levels appear adequate.

One might considerably affect their vitamin D level by their financial status. Access to safe outdoor spaces, foods high in vitamin D, and supplements is set by social level. Some groups suffer "vitamin D deserts," in which case socioeconomic or environmental restrictions complicate obtaining enough vitamin D.

Food poverty can affect vitamin D level as some of the best dietary sources—like fatty fish—can be expensive. To assist to address these gaps, public health campaigns are looking at community education and fortification programs.

[Economic Impact: Low-income groups show up to 50% more prevalence of vitamin D shortage.]

For colleges and universities, maintaining optimal vitamin D levels among staff members and students poses unique challenges. Vitamin D levels vary depending on early morning schedules, less outside activities, and more time spent inside.

New delivery techniques including topical therapies, time-released formulations, and even clothing boosted in vitamin D content are under investigation by researchers. Smart buildings might use UV-transparent materials allowing good UVB rays while restricting harmful radiation.

[Future Tech: Within the next decade wearable devices might let us check vitamin D levels real-time.]

Vitamin D is essentially a big paradox in modern health: a molecule so essential our bodies can produce with just sunshine but so elusive that over a billion people worldwide suffer from insufficient levels. Unlike any other vitamin, D is a hormone and a nutrient that coordinates several distinct biological activity all over our body. This element is among the most fascinating and crucial ones for human health given its unique dual character and should get especially attention in our modern world.

Our tour of vitamin D reveals its remarkable distribution inside the human body. From preserving strong teeth and bones to boosting immunological function, from enhancing physical performance to regulating mood, vitamin D's effects go much beyond what we initially realized. The knowledge of the importance of vitamin D changed when we realized practically every type of cell in our body had vitamin D receptors. Not only is it about avoiding rickets now; vitamin D is crucial for everything, including DNA repair and brain activity.

Maintaining appropriate amounts of vitamin D provides formerly unheard-of challenges in modern life. Together with more screen time and less outside activity, our indoor lifestyle has fundamentally disrupted our natural vitamin D production. Urban life adds a another degree of challenge since tall buildings produce "vitamin D shadows" and air pollution filters vital UVB rays. Though very important for preventing skin cancer, our well-intentioned sun protection habits may inadvertently lead to vitamin D inadequacy.

Distinct populations have distinct problems with vitamin D. The elderly often suffer from a lack as their skin naturally produces less vitamin D. Darker skinned persons need more sun to produce the same degree of vitamin D as those with lighter skin. People from northern latitudes, shift workers, and office workers all have unique set of challenges. Pregnant women and growing children have additional needs; athletes require optimal levels for greatest performance.

Vitamin D levels have effects on health well beyond merely bone strength. Research is continually revealing fresh uses for this vitamin in immune system, mental health, physical performance, and sickness prevention. From respiratory infections to autoimmune diseases, low vitamin D levels have been linked to increased risk of several diseases. The COVID-19 outbreak underscored the significance vitamin D plays in immune system and its need in modern health problems.

Maintaining optimal vitamin D levels requires a complex understanding of several factors. Seasonal fluctuations affect our natural vitamin D synthesis; in many places, winter months particularly cause problems. Although helpful, dietary sources might prove insufficient on their own. The needs for supplements are much influenced by personal traits including age, weight, skin tone, and lifestyle. The trick is to find the perfect blend of sun exposure, diet, and supplements for every person's individual situation.

Research on vitamin D is still in progress. New technologies to monitor and optimize vitamin D level are under development. Customized approaches based on personal situation and genetic profiles have promise. More than ever, vitamin D is vital as its role in preventing and regulating modern health problems draws more attention.

Environmental factors are becoming more and more important for our vitamin D status. Preserving optimal levels is challenging with changing lifestyles, air pollution, and climate change as well. Some original ideas are beginning to arise from new supplement delivery methods to vitamin D-friendly building design. Understanding these challenges helps us to design better strategies to maintain appropriate levels.

Based on understanding of vitamin D, one realistically need a diversified approach. Regular monitoring, approach change depending on seasonal fluctuations, attention to co-factor magnesium and vitamin K2, and understanding of personal risk factors all play very essential roles. Many times, success comes from combining many strategies: smart sun exposure, dietary choices, and appropriate supplementation when needed.

As our research of vitamin D comes to a close, its importance in human health becomes ever more clear. This vitamin connects us in strange ways to our environment, our development, and modern challenges. Whether from diet, sunlight, or supplements, maintaining appropriate vitamin D levels is still rather essential for health in our modern surroundings. Our understanding of this incredible vitamin will only increase as research progresses and new challenges arise; so, it is even more important as one of the key predictor of human health.

ΔΔΔ

E FOR ESSENTIAL

Let us now meet vitamin E, your body's primary defense against cell damage. Though most people know vitamin E from cosmetic products, its value transcends looks.

Vitamin E is special among the key fat-soluble antioxidants in your body. While vitamin C protects the watery parts of your cells, vitamin E retains the fatty regions including cell membranes and brain tissue. It's like having a waterproof coating protecting your most delicate cell parts from damage. These fatty areas are more prone to oxidative damage, which can lead to early aging and other health issues, so this protection is highly crucial.

Finding vitamin E seems like a scientific detective story. Rats fed rancid fat were found unable to be able to breed, researchers discovered in 1922. Returning some oils fixed the problem and led to the discovery of this essential vitamin. Today, we understand that vitamin E is not only important for reproduction but also for brain function, immune system operation, skin integrity, and even athletic performance.

Modern life provides particular challenges for vitamin E levels. Although processed food often lack this element, growing environmental pollutants and stress create increased demand for antioxidant protection. Like living in a city with more crime, you need additional security. Fortunately, nature loads vitamin E in many foods from nuts and seeds to leafy greens and certain oils.

[Power Fact: Vitamin E may kill free radicals up to 200 times quicker than many other antioxidants, your body's quick reaction squad against cellular harm.]

View vitamin E as your internal preservation mechanism. As antioxidants stop food from rotting, vitamin E helps your cells from the inside out not "rusting". Particularly depending on this protection are active persons, those living in polluted surroundings, and everyone striving to retain young vitality.

Given its high fat content and great use of oxygen, vitamin E's protective qualities notably help your brain.

[Some studies suggest that as we age, vitamin E levels may help to maintain cognitive performance.]

The way vitamin E works is fascinating. When a free radical (think of it as a cellular vandal) tries to damage a cell membrane, vitamin E steps in and takes the hit instead. But here's the clever part - vitamin E doesn't become useless after neutralizing a threat. It can be recycled by other antioxidants, particularly vitamin C, making it an incredibly efficient defense system.

Let's explore how particularly vitamin E excels in terms of brain performance. Your brain is around 60%

fat, hence it is particularly vulnerable to oxidative damage, just like a high-performance computer needs particular protection. Vitamin E protects these sensitive fatty cells from damage that would affect everything from memory to mood.

Recent research reveal areas of the brain connected to learning and memory concentrate vitamin E. Your body seems to know just where to set its strongest defenses. As vitamin E levels drop, these areas might actually start to show higher susceptibility to age-related degradation. Maintaining appropriate vitamin E levels seems to help preserve cognitive abilities as we age; think of this as type of brain insurance for your golden years.

Here's where it gets very interesting: vitamin E not only protects but also increases the communication capacity of your brain cells. It maintains the integrity of neural membranes, therefore allowing brain cells to more successfully send information. This increased communication might help to explain why some studies found faster response times and more mental sharpness linked with better vitamin E levels.

Students and sportsmen pay heed; the preservation of vitamin E covers performance. Mental weariness may have some relationship with brain oxidative stress after considerable study or training. Enough vitamin E can keep you cognitively active for longer periods of time and counteract this stress.

[Brain Fact: Your brain uses about 20% of the oxygen your body absorbs even though just 2% of your weight. This high oxygen consumption makes brain tissue more vulnerable to oxidative damage - exactly what vitamin E helps prevent.]

Vitamin E and brain function are closely related early in life. Enough vitamin E both throughout pregnancy and early infancy determines appropriate brain development. This early protection provides the groundwork for lifetime brain health, much as building a house with the best materials from the foundation up.

[Protection Note: Studies show optimal levels may help slow down the process of brain aging even if vitamin E cannot halt all of it. Higher vitamin E levels have some studies suggesting to up to 25% better cognitive preservation in aged adults.]

Modern living offers unique challenges for brain preservation. Stress, environmental toxins, even our reliance on technology might increase the need of our brain for antioxidant protection. Think of it as needing more defense in a more crowded, stressful environment on buses.

One of the most strong antioxidants available in nature, vitamin E continuously protects your body from damage inside cells. Unlike simpler nutrients, it is a family of eight compounds: four tocopherols and four tocotrienols, each with particular protective ability for your body. Though the most well-known form is alpha-tocopherol, its seven siblings also aid to maintain health and halt damage all over your body.

One rather amazing cardiovascular benefit of vitamin E is acting as the maintenance crew for your blood vessels, it maintains vessels flexible and healthy and helps to prevent cholesterol oxidation. Vitamin E neutralizes the free radicals generated by the motion of your heart, so reaching your heart muscle itself. Some studies show that by up to 40%, sufficient vitamin E levels may reduce cardiovascular risk, which is really amazing in our modern society with rising issues with heart health.

Vitamin E is absolutely vital for optimum immune system performance. It helps your body to manage inflammatory reactions all around and raises immune cell activity. As we become older, when our immune systems naturally begin to decline, this becomes rather important. Especially in its gamma-tocopherol form, vitamin E's anti-inflammatory properties help reduce too much inflammation that could worsen certain chronic conditions.

The benefits of vitamin E for skin go well beyond its usual use in cosmetics. Approaches from the inside out, it provides essential protection against environmental pressures as UV damage and pollutants. This inside protection might assist to maintain moisture levels, reduce scarring, and promote skin healing. These benefits become much more apparent when combined with other nutrients such as vitamin C, thereby creating a whole system for maintaining skin integrity and attractiveness.

The modern lifestyle creates before unheard-of need for vitamin E protection. Environmental contaminants, processed food, high levels of stress itself, and increased screen time all contribute to higher oxidative stress in our bodies. Fortunately, nature provides several sources of this essential vitamin. Natural forms of vitamin E abound in nuts, seeds, vegetable oils, green leafy vegetables, all containing the whole range of tocopherols and tocotrienols.

Special populations demand extra cautious attention to vitamin E level. Pregnant women require it for healthy fetal development; athletes need more for recovery and performance; and older people may benefit from increased intake for immunological and cognitive support. Those with digestive issues might have to pay more attention to absorption; smokers typically require extra vitamin E to combat increased oxidative stress.

Although daily demands for vitamin E seem low—about 15mg for adults—meting these needs with a balanced diet has advantages not generally available from pills. Food sources both complement other nutrients to increase their efficacy and offer the entire spectrum of vitamin E components. Moreover, the body normally absorbs and utilizes natural forms of vitamin E far more efficiently than synthetic equivalents.

Understanding the purpose of vitamin E opens fascinating chances to maximize wellness. From supporting cardiovascular health to enhancing immunological function, from safeguarding skin to sustaining cognitive capacity, this flexible vitamin is necessary everywhere in the body. Maintaining optimal vitamin E level becomes even more crucial as research highlight new effects and ways of action.

Particularly interesting is the way vitamin E interacts with your brain. Being 60% fat, your brain notably benefits from vitamin E's fat-soluble antioxidant properties. Concentrates of vitamin E in regions connected to memory and learning serve to protect these vital areas from oxidative damage. Studies suggest that maintaining suitable vitamin E levels helps preserve cognitive performance and maybe slow down age-related mental decline.

The sports world recognizes increasingly the importance of vitamin E for performance and recovery. Your body produces more free radicals during severe exercise, hence you need more protection from antioxidants. Ideal vitamin E levels help athletes to recover faster and reduce muscular injury. Vitamin E protects both physical and mental function by helping battle oxidative damage brought on by exercise in both muscles and brain tissue.

Appropriate vitamin E levels improve women's

health rather dramatically. From comfort during menstruation to reproductive health, vitamin E is really vital all through a woman's life. When pregnant, it encourages fetal growth—especially that of the brain and nervous system development. As women get older, vitamin E's antioxidant properties might help ease menopausal symptoms and increase general energy.

Given environmental concerns, vitamin E is more vital than it has ever been. Rising with air pollution, UV radiation, and other environmental contaminants is our bodies' need for antioxidant protection. Urbanites might need extra attention to their vitamin E level as city life generally involves higher contact to pollutants and oxidative stressors.

Still another significant benefit of vitamin E is illness prevention. Studies show suitable levels helping to reduce chances of several ailments, including certain kinds of cancer and cataracts. Although its antioxidant properties protect against cellular damage that could support the growth of diseases, its anti-inflammatory properties might assist regulate chronic conditions.

The digestive tract greatly affects how much vitamin E is absorbed. E absorbs best from dietary fat, much like other fat-soluble vitamins. Those on low-fat diets or with digestive issues could not get all the benefits from their vitamin E intake. Understanding this enables one to see why whole food sources—which typically include natural fats—have better vitamin E absorption than manufactured tablets.

[Essential Note: The protective network produced by the interactions of any one vitamin E type or other nutrient is far less strong than this. This clarifies the reason dietary sources often provide more benefits than single supplements.]

Let us break down how best to optimize your daily, sensible vitamin E intake. Although the recommended daily dose for adults is 15mg, depending on your lifestyle, degree of stress, and health conditions your personal needs may vary substantially. Modern life poses particular difficulties on our vitamin E demands, with factors like air pollution, stress, and processed foods maybe pushing our needs above the prescribed amounts.

Nature packs vitamin E in some foods with incredible efficiency. With up to 7.4mg per ounce, almonds and sunflower seeds particularly serve to provide the best sources from nuts and seeds. Leafy greens like spinach and Swiss chard complement vitamin E in terms of minerals that boost its absorption and efficacy. Among the healthy fats from sources that not only provide vitamin E but also help to maximize absorption of it from other foods are avocados and olive oil.

Timing and balance of vitamin E consumption are really significant. Eating meals high in vitamin E together with some good fat considerably boosts absorption as they are fat-soluble. It might be especially beneficial as early intake provides antioxidant protection throughout day when environmental stressors are highest. Combining foods strong in vitamin E with sources of vitamin C has a synergistic effect that enhances the protective properties of both elements.

Cooking methods and storage can greatly affect the vitamin E concentration in foods. Heat and light may degrade vitamin E, so suitable storage of nuts, seeds, and oils becomes fairly crucial. Light cooking methods as steaming or rapid stir-frying maintain more vitamin E than long, high-heat cooking. Generally speaking, fresh, well preserved foods have more vitamin E than those held for long periods of time or subjected to too much light and heat.

One should particularly pay close attention to absorption factors. Vitamin E absorption can be lowered by low-fat diets, certain medications, and digestive issues as well. Maximizing absorption calls for dealing with complete food sources and ensuring one gets adequate good fat. Some people—especially those with digestive issues or greater needs—may find tremendous advantage from targeted supplements under physician supervision.

Athletes and active adults may have to pay particular attention to their vitamin E intake. Exercise increases oxidative stress of the body, so maybe increasing demand for vitamin E. Strategic eating both before and after workouts can help reduce oxidative damage caused by exercise and promote recovery. For individuals who exercise intensely or endurance athletes, this becomes very vital.

Interactions of vitamin E with other nutrients create a complex network. It works very well with selenium, vitamin C, and other antioxidants notably. Understanding these interactions helps one to realize why, with their natural nutritional combinations, whole food sources usually provide better benefits than individual medicines. This combined effect underlines the requirement of a varied, nutrient-dense diet over simple supplementation.

[Practical Note: Instead of depending simply on tablets, try to integrate a variety of foods high in vitamin E into your daily diet. The natural combination of nutrients in whole foods provides benefits not generally achievable from single supplements.]

The more we learn about the purposes of vitamin E, its importance in different periods of life becomes very clear. Especially in the growth of the brain and nervous system, vitamin E becomes quite important during pregnancy. Appropriate dosages strengthen the immune system of the developing baby and help avoid various pregnancy complications. By protecting reproductive cells from oxidative damage and hence encouraging hormonal balance, vitamin E might benefit women trying to conceive.

Another group with especially low vitamin E intake are athletes. During a strenuous exercise, oxidative stress increases dramatically all over the body. Vitamin E may speed recovery time and protect muscle cells from damage caused by exercise between training sessions. Studies reveal that athletes with optimal vitamin E levels experienced less muscle discomfort and quicker recovery times; yet, timing and dosage should be carefully examined to maximize benefits without sacrificing training adaptations.

Growing older begs special inquiries regarding vitamin E levels. As we age, our bodies progressively lose their ability to fight oxidative stress; so, antioxidant protection becomes even more crucial. Given studies show vitamin E may help elderly people keep memory and learning ability, its relevance in cognitive function becomes rather important. Given that age inevitably impairs the immune system, its maintenance of immunological function becomes also rather important.

Environmental factors are causing changes in our vitamin E demands. Given its exposure to pollution, electromagnetic radiation, and other environmental challenges, urban living might increase our need for antioxidant defense. The vitamin E content of our food is influenced by modern farming techniques and climate change; so, wise dietary choices become even more important. People who live in extremely polluted areas or work in high-stress environments might have to concentrate particularly on their vitamin E intake.

Studies are exposing continually shifting relationships between vitamin E and the prevention of chronic illnesses. Its anti-inflammatory properties might enable management of conditions ranging from arthritis to asthma. Although additional research is required to fully grasp these relationships, several studies suggest suitable vitamin E levels might help reduce the risk of certain cancers and heart diseases. Not quick fixes, consistent, long-term optimal levels seem to be the solution.

The demands of modern life put especially on our vitamin E level certain stress. While processed foods occasionally lack vitamin E, extended screen time produces oxidative stress in our eyes and brain. Environmental toxins, inadequate sleep, and chronic stress all increase the demand for antioxidant defense in our body. Understanding these modern problems helps us to choose, wisely, dietary and supplementary course of action.

Including vitamin E into daily life demands both awareness of its benefits and limitations. Though there are many of medicines, food still is the best source of vitamin E. This complete package approach has more benefits than individual supplements especially for long-term health maintenance.

One must know absorption factors if one wants optimum usage of vitamin E. Correct absorption depends on dietary fat, hence natural fat content in nuts and seeds makes them excellent sources. Timing is also important; consuming foods strong in vitamin E together with meals heavy in healthy fats dramatically boosts absorption. Those seeking protection against daily environmental stressors notably benefit from morning use.

New research reveals remarkable link between vitamin E and genetic expression. Especially those connected to inflammation and antioxidant protection, this vitamin seems to regulate the activation of specific genes. This genetic interaction implies that, based on genetic profiles, future vitamin E recommendations might become more customized since it helps explain why some people could benefit more from optimal vitamin E levels than others.

Given our environment focused on fitness, the relationship between vitamin E and exercise draws especially attention. Vitamin E protects cell membranes against oxidative damage brought on by intense exercise. Timing is also crucial; some research suggest that high-dose vitamin E given just before exercise may actually inhibit certain positive effects. The answer is to maintain appropriate baseline levels by diet rather than highly potent supplements.

Environmental pollutants and modern living choices are influencing our vitamin E demands as well. Under screen time, air pollution, processed meals, and constant stress, our bodies start to oxidize more. Particularly urban living impairs our antioxidant defenses, so intentional vitamin E intake becomes even more important. Those who live under severe stress or in cities might have to concentrate specifically on their vitamin E level by adjusting their diet and way of living.

Customized approaches will help to guide vitamin E research further. These days, scientists examine how specific factors like heredity, lifestyle, and environmental exposure influence vitamin E needs. This study suggests moving from one-size-fits-all guidance toward more intricate, customized guidelines. Understanding these unique variations helps one to realize why some persons can benefit more from increased vitamin E intake than others. [Modern Note: As new environmental pressures and lifestyle components continually revealing new uses for the protective properties of vitamin E, this nutrient is growing in importance in our modern culture.]

Particularly in relation to modern health concerns, our understanding of vitamin E is always evolving. Recent investigations reveal its probable role in disorders including neurodegenerative illnesses, autoimmune diseases, and metabolic syndrome. The key is not just in pills but also in optimizing the body's absorption of this vitamin by means of all-encompassing diet and lifestyle practices.

Emerging technologies are changing our approaches of monitoring vitamin E level optimization. Wearable technology detecting oxidative stress levels might soon allow individuals increase their vitamin E consumption according on real-time physiological demands instead of depending on general recommendations. This technical advancement points to more specialized vitamin E enhancing strategies at a time.

The effect of the gut flora on vitamin E absorption and use is another frontier under research. Modern scientists know that some gut bacteria influence our absorption and use efficiency for vitamin E. This understanding opens new chances to maximize vitamin E level by means of probiotic supplements and dietary adjustments promoting beneficial gut flora. The interaction between gut health and vitamin

E efficiency might assist to explain why some people respond differently to equal ingestion levels.

Environmental problems keep driving our unexpected vitamin E requirements. Beyond well-known stresses like UV radiation and pollution, microplastics and electromagnetic radiation might increase our demand for antioxidant defense. Climate change affects the vitamin E level in our food sources as well as our exposure to environmental pressures; thus, intentional dietary choices become even more important.

Vitamins E combined with other minerals reveals complex cooperative relationships. While vitamin E is more effective when vitamin C helps recycle it, other nutrients such selenium and CoQ10 work with vitamin E to provide whole cellular protection. Understanding these connections enables one to see why whole food approaches frequently show more success than isolated supplements. Knowing and maximizing these nutritional interactions will most likely assist to define vitamin E optimization moving ahead.

Long-term health maintenance grounded on vitamin E optimization requires a combination approach. The main focus should be on maintaining appropriate levels rather than maximum consumption using consistent, food-based strategies enhanced as required. This approach recognizes that more is not necessarily better; too much vitamin E supplements may potentially offset some of its expected advantages. The trick is to get the right balance for your needs and circumstances.

[Future Focus: As research highlight new roles for vitamin E, its importance in preventive medicine methods grows. One must first grasp personal factors impacting vitamin E demands if one is to maximize health.]

With growing interest in supplements, understanding of the safety profile of vitamin E becomes rather important. While natural foods seldom ever cause problems, high-dose supplements should be used with great care. The upper limit for adults is 1,000 mg daily, even if many physicians suggest staying well below this dose unless specifically advised. Too many supplements might interfere with blood coagulation, especially in those on blood-thinning medications.

Especially in the treatment of chronic disorders, therapeutic applications of vitamin E keep expanding. In neurological illnesses, cardiovascular disease, some types of cancer, optimised vitamin E levels show promising effects. Still, time and amount are really crucial; some disorders respond better to specific forms of vitamin E or combinations with other nutrients. This complexity emphasizes the requirement of professional leadership in the treatment of vitamin E.

The role of vitamin E in skin condition and beauty

goes beyond common knowledge. While exterior treatments offer benefits, for skin condition interior optimization is very important. From inside, vitamin E supports collagen production, inflammation reduction, and oxidative damage protection of skin cells. Combining internal and outside therapies typically yields excellent results for skin health and anti-aging benefits.

Athletes and individuals who like fitness require specific consideration in vitamin E plans. High-intensity exercise increases oxidative stress, thereby perhaps quickly lowering vitamin E levels. Studies show, meantime, that excessively high antioxidant supplements might interfere with training adaptations. The secret is careful timing: avoid high-dose supplements just before training sessions and preserve optimal baseline levels by diet.

Modern environmental concerns offer vitamin E status considerable importance. Beyond advised levels, usage of digital gadgets, aircraft travel, and environmental toxins might increase our vitamin E demands. Those with high-stress occupations, frequent travelers, and urbanites may benefit from more targeted vitamin E optimization strategies. This modern environment begs a reconsideration of accepted dosing guidelines.

Drug interactions involving vitamin E call special attention. Common medications include several blood thinners and drugs lowering cholesterol can interact with vitamin E supplements. Moreover, several medical conditions might affect vitamin E absorption or consumption. This complexity emphasizes the importance of professional assistance in regard to supplements, particularly for those on regular medication or with present medical problems.

The topography of vitamin E research is continually shifting and interesting new discoveries abound. New delivery techniques under investigation by researchers might right now increase absorption and effectiveness. For example, nanoencapsulation technology shows promise in raising the bioavailability of vitamin E, thereby maybe making lesser dosages more advantageous. Especially for those with absorption issues, this discovery might change our perspective on vitamin E supplementation.

Studies on age-related aspects reveal even more important roles for vitamin E in normal aging. Apart from its clear benefits for brain function, current studies suggest vitamin E may influence genes related to cellular aging mechanisms and lifespan. Particularly interesting prospects come from the interaction between vitamin E and telomeres, the protective caps covering our chromosomes. Some research indicate that increasing vitamin E level might help to maintain telomere length, therefore influencing our cell aging process.

The relationship between vitamin E and immune

system resilience becomes even more important in a post-pandemic setting. Enough vitamin E, according to studies, can increase the effectiveness of immunizations and support the body in fighting illnesses. Especially for older people and those with compromised immune systems, this becomes fairly crucial. Vitamin E optimization seems to have a timing; maintaining suitable levels before immunological problems demonstrates greater success than adding later on.

The impacts of climate change on vitamin E content in foods generate new challenges necessitating innovative solutions. Agricultural researchers are developing crop varieties with greater vitamin E while food experts consider preservation methods to maintain vitamin E levels throughout processing and storage. Knowing these challenges directs not just specific diets but also more broad public health initiatives.

Personalized medical approaches to boost vitamin E will be the next step. These days, genetic testing can discover variations in how people absorb and use vitamin E, which could help to explain why some people receive more from pills than others. Depending on human genetic profiles, environmental exposures, and health condition, this knowledge directs more specific recommendations.

[Future Vision: Artificial intelligence analyzing vitamin E needs could someday provide real-time, tailored recommendations based on numerous parameters including activity level, environmental exposure, and genetic predisposition.]

Modern studies are revealing how vitamin E operates in epigenetics—that is, how our genes express themselves in response to environmental cues. This vitamin apparently affects patterns of gene expression linked to inflammation, disease resistance, and aging. This knowledge creates new opportunities for tailored diets where ideal vitamin E levels can help change genetic predispositions to various disease problems.

Long-term vitamin E health maintenance calls both knowledge of its advantages and drawbacks. Although poor nations still have low rates of deficiency, suboptimal levels are very widespread and might cause numerous health problems. Not to maximize consumption; rather, the aim is to maintain steady, ideal levels by meals and, if needed, specific supplements. Usually, this all-around strategy proves to be more successful than intensive supplement programs.

As our food supply gets increasingly complicated, quality issues become ever more important. Growing circumstances, storage environment, and processing technique all greatly affect the food vitamin E concentration. Particularly in their natural forms, organic vegetables generally include more vitamin E. Knowing these elements helps one to choose foods and supplements in keeping with knowledge.

Particularly special populations should pay great attention to vitamin E levels. To optimize vitamin E, pregnant women, elderly people, athletes, and those with chronic medical problems might need alternative strategies. More regular monitoring and modified therapies depending on their particular need and situation help these groups greatly.

[Final Thought: Beyond its simple antioxidant action, vitamin E is quite valuable for human health. Studies reveal fresh roles and linkages, therefore this vitamin becomes more and more important for ideal health in our current environment.]

To sum up, made up of eight molecules, four

tocopherols and four tocotrienols, vitamin E is among the most evolved antioxidant systems found in nature. Together, each member of this vitamin family provides unique protective qualities to your body, therefore creating a whole protection mechanism against cellular damage. The primary fat-soluble antioxidant, vitamin E shines notably in protecting cell membranes, brain tissue, and other fat-rich areas of your body from oxidative damage.

Modern existence brings until unheard-of demand for vitamin E protection. Environmental pollutants, digital device radiation, processed meals, and chronic stress all affect our need for antioxidant defense. Especially urban living presents unique challenges requiring strict attention to vitamin E status.

Together with low vitamin E concentration in many foods, these modern demands make intentional optimization of vitamin E consumption even more important.

The benefits of optimal vitamin E level go well beyond mere prevention of oxidative damage. Research underline its crucial relevance in immune system support, athletic performance, cardiovascular health, and cognitive function. Vitamin E could possibly influence our aging process, helping retain skin health, and maintains appropriate gene expression. Its ability to traverse the blood-brain barrier makes it particularly crucial for maintaining neural tissue; its presence in cell membranes all over the body aids in preservation of cellular integrity.

Nature packs vitamin E especially in some meals for good reason. Especially almonds, sunflower seeds, leafy greens, avocados, and certain oils provide not just vitamin E but also the complementing nutrients and excellent fats required for optimum absorption. This natural packaging demonstrates more efficiency than single supplements as the full nutritional profile helps better absorption and usage.

Special populations need specifically for particular consideration of vitamin E level. Older folks benefit from its cognitive protection; athletes require more for performance and recovery; and pregnant women need it for fetal development. Urbanites incur increased oxidative stress while those with digestive issues may find it difficult to absorb. Understanding these specific needs helps one create well-defined strategies for various realms of life.

The path of vitamin E optimization is toward always personalized solutions. These days, genetic testing can discover variations in how people absorb and utilize vitamin E, which could help to explain why some people gain more from increased use than others. Although knowledge of environmental effects helps create more efficient preventative strategies, new delivery systems and monitoring technologies seem to guarantee more accurate optimization.

Success with vitamin E requires for a reasonable, informed approach. Using consistent, well-planned strategies, maintaining appropriate levels should take front stage rather than maximum consumption. Knowing personal needs, environmental challenges, and lifestyle choices helps one create reasonable plans for long-term health maintenance. Studies exposing new roles and links highlight the significance of vitamin E in modern health.

△△△

VITAMIN MYTHS EXPOSED

Vitamins are essential for maintaining good health, but with so much conflicting information out there, it's easy to get lost in the myths and misconceptions surrounding them. From claims of miracle cures to the overhyped benefits of certain supplements, the world of vitamins can be confusing. In this chapter, we'll separate fact from fiction, debunking common vitamin myths, and shedding light on what's really backed by science. Whether you're looking to improve your diet or enhance your overall wellness, understanding the truth behind these vitamins is key to making informed decisions about your health.

Myth: You can't overdose on vitamins because they're natural.

Fact: Fat-soluble vitamins (A, D, E, K) can accumulate to toxic levels.

Myth: More vitamins means better health.

Fact: Excessive supplementation can interfere with nutrient balance and potentially harm health.

Myth: All vitamin supplements are created equal.

Fact: Quality, absorption rates, and formulations

vary significantly between products. Natural forms often have better absorption and come with complementary nutrients.

Myth: If you eat well, you don't need to worry about vitamins.

Fact: Modern farming practices, stress, and environmental factors can increase vitamin needs beyond what diet alone provides.

Myth: Vitamin C prevents colds.

Fact: While it doesn't prevent colds, it may reduce their duration and severity.

Myth: Natural vitamins are always better than synthetic ones.

Fact: What matters most is bioavailability and proper formulation. Some synthetic vitamins are equally effective.

Myth: You need to take supplements every day.

Fact: A balanced diet often provides sufficient vitamins for healthy individuals.

Myth: Vitamins provide energy.

Fact: Vitamins don't provide energy directly; they help your body convert food into energy.

Myth: Take vitamins on an empty stomach for best absorption.

Fact: Many vitamins need food, especially fats, for proper absorption.

Myth: Morning is the only good time to take vitamins.

Fact: Timing depends on the specific vitamin and your daily routine.

Myth: Vitamins work immediately.

Fact: Most vitamins need consistent intake over time to show benefits.

Myth: You can't overdose on water-soluble vitamins.

Fact: While less common, excessive intake of water-soluble vitamins can cause problems.

Myth: Crushing vitamins makes them work better.

Fact: Some vitamins are specifically formulated for timed release and shouldn't be crushed.

Myth: All vitamin content is lost during cooking.

Fact: Some vitamins become more bioavailable through cooking.

Myth: Fresh fruits always have more vitamins than frozen.

Fact: Frozen fruits often retain more vitamins as they're frozen at peak ripeness.

Myth: Raw vegetables always provide more vitamins.

Fact: Some vitamins become more available through cooking (like lycopene in tomatoes).

Myth: Juicing is the best way to get vitamins.

Fact: Whole fruits and vegetables often provide better vitamin absorption due to fiber content.

Myth: White vegetables have no vitamins.

Fact: Many white vegetables are rich in various vitamins and nutrients.

Myth: All vitamin pills are effective in the same way.

Fact: The form, dose, and quality of the supplement impact its effectiveness.

Myth: If a vitamin supplement is labeled "natural," it must be better.

Fact: "Natural" doesn't necessarily mean safer or more effective. The source and form of the vitamin matter.

Myth: Vitamin D is only important for bone health.

Fact: Vitamin D also supports immune function,

mood regulation, and heart health.

Myth: Taking extra vitamin E will prevent heart disease.

Fact: There's no clear evidence that extra vitamin E prevents heart disease, and excessive amounts may cause harm.

Myth: Prenatal vitamins are only for pregnant women.

Fact: Prenatal vitamins are high in folic acid and iron, which can benefit anyone, not just pregnant women.

Myth: All vitamins are absorbed the same way.

Fact: Fat-soluble vitamins need fat for absorption, while water-soluble vitamins are absorbed with water.

Myth: You can get all your vitamins from food alone.

Fact: Some individuals may need supplements due to specific health conditions, lifestyle factors, or nutrient absorption issues.

Myth: Vitamin B12 can be absorbed from plant-based foods.

Fact: Vitamin B12 is primarily found in animal products; vegetarians and vegans may need supplements or fortified foods.

Myth: Vitamin A from supplements is better than from food.

Fact: Beta-carotene (found in fruits and vegetables)

is safer and better absorbed than high-dose synthetic vitamin A.

Myth: Vitamin K only helps with blood clotting.

Fact: Vitamin K also plays a role in bone health and cardiovascular health.

Myth: Vitamin supplements can replace a poor diet.

Fact: Supplements are meant to supplement a healthy diet, not replace it.

Myth: All vitamin D is the same.

Fact: Vitamin D2 and D3 are not identical; vitamin D3 is more effective at raising vitamin D levels in the body.

Myth: Taking a high dose of vitamin C can cure a cold.

Fact: High doses of vitamin C won't cure a cold, but may reduce its severity and duration.

Myth: Vitamin B6 can improve your mood.

Fact: While B6 supports brain function, there's no strong evidence it can treat mood disorders like depression.

Myth: Vitamin B12 deficiency is rare.

Fact: Vitamin B12 deficiency is more common than you think, especially in older adults, vegetarians, and people with absorption issues.

Myth: Vitamin A is toxic at high doses, but only if it's synthetic.

Fact: Both synthetic and natural sources of vitamin A can be toxic at high doses, especially in pregnant women.

Myth: Vitamin supplements can help you lose weight.

Fact: No vitamin supplement has been proven to directly cause weight loss; healthy diet and exercise are key.

Myth: You can't get enough vitamin D if you live in a cold climate.

Fact: Even in colder climates, you can get enough vitamin D from sunlight or supplements if needed.

Myth: Eating more citrus fruits is the best way to get vitamin C.

Fact: Many non-citrus fruits and vegetables (like bell peppers and strawberries) provide even more vitamin

C.

Myth: Vitamin C will protect you from sunburn.

Fact: Vitamin C can help with skin health but doesn't replace sunscreen or protect against UV radiation.

Myth: Biotin can make your hair grow faster.

Fact: Biotin deficiency can lead to hair loss, but if you're not deficient, biotin supplementation won't speed up hair growth.

Myth: Vitamin D is only important in the winter.

Fact: Vitamin D is essential year-round; regular sun exposure or supplementation is necessary, even in warmer months.

Myth: Vitamin E is only good for your skin.

Fact: Vitamin E is also crucial for immune function, eye health, and cellular repair.

Myth: Vitamin B12 is only needed by vegetarians and vegans.

Fact: Vitamin B12 deficiency can affect anyone, especially older adults and people with absorption issues.

Myth: You can only get vitamin D from the sun.

Fact: Vitamin D can also be obtained from foods like fortified milk, fatty fish, and supplements.

Myth: Eating a lot of carrots will improve your night vision.

Fact: While carrots are rich in beta-carotene (a source of vitamin A), they won't give you superhuman vision.

Myth: Vitamin C can protect you from all forms of cancer.

Fact: While vitamin C supports immune function, it does not prevent or cure cancer.

Myth: You need to take multiple supplements to get all the vitamins.

Fact: Many multivitamins contain a wide range of essential vitamins and minerals, but your body may need specific ones depending on your diet and health.

Myth: Taking more vitamin C will prevent you from

getting sick.

Fact: Vitamin C can boost immune function but doesn't guarantee immunity from illness.

Myth: All vitamin D supplements are the same.

Fact: Vitamin D3 is more effective than D2 for raising blood levels of vitamin D.

Myth: You should take high doses of vitamin C when you're sick.

Fact: While vitamin C may shorten the duration of colds, it won't cure them.

Myth: Vitamin B12 injections are always better than oral supplements.

Fact: Oral vitamin B12 supplements are just as

effective for most people as injections, unless there are absorption issues.

Myth: You only need vitamins if you're sick or tired.

Fact: Vitamins are important for maintaining general health, energy, and overall well-being.

Myth: If you eat foods rich in vitamins, you don't need supplements.

Fact: Some people may still need supplements due to health conditions, medications, or dietary restrictions.

Myth: Your body stores water-soluble vitamins like it does fat-soluble ones.

Fact: Water-soluble vitamins (e.g., B vitamins and

vitamin C) are not stored in the body and must be replenished regularly.

Myth: You can't overdose on vitamin B12.

Fact: While it's rare, excessive intake of B12 can cause side effects like skin rashes or problems with nerve function.

Myth: Supplements are the best way to get vitamins.

Fact: Whole foods are always a better source of vitamins, as they provide fiber and other beneficial nutrients.

Myth: Vitamin A is only found in animal products.

Fact: Plant-based foods like carrots and sweet potatoes provide beta-carotene, which the body converts to vitamin A.

Myth: A daily multivitamin will cover all your nutritional needs.

Fact: Multivitamins can fill gaps, but they can't replace a healthy, balanced diet.

Myth: Vitamin K is only important for blood clotting.

Fact: Vitamin K also plays a role in bone health and the prevention of osteoporosis.

Myth: Vitamin B3 (Niacin) can lower cholesterol significantly.

Fact: While niacin can help lower cholesterol, it should be taken under medical supervision as high doses can cause serious side effects.

Myth: Vitamin D is only important for bone health.

Fact: Vitamin D also plays a role in immune health, mood regulation, and the prevention of chronic diseases.

Myth: Taking high doses of vitamin B5 will help with acne.

Fact: While vitamin B5 supports skin health, there's no evidence that high doses will treat acne.

Myth: You need to take vitamins in pill form to get their benefits.

Fact: Many vitamins can be consumed in food sources like fruits, vegetables, and fortified foods.

Myth: Vitamin B12 is absorbed better through sublingual supplements.

Fact: Sublingual B12 may have a slight advantage for some people, but it's not necessary for most.

Myth: Vitamin E is the cure for wrinkles.

Fact: While vitamin E helps protect skin from damage, there's no magic pill for reversing wrinkles.

Myth: High-dose vitamin A is good for acne.

Fact: High-dose vitamin A can be toxic and should only be used under medical supervision.

Myth: Vitamin C will cure a hangover.

Fact: Vitamin C won't cure a hangover, but staying hydrated and replenishing electrolytes may help.

Myth: Vitamin C increases your iron absorption.

Fact: Vitamin C helps enhance the absorption of non-heme iron from plant sources.

Myth: Vitamin B12 is found in all plant-based foods.

Fact: Vitamin B12 is naturally found only in animal products, so vegans need fortified foods or supplements.

Myth: Vitamin D is unnecessary if you eat enough dairy.

Fact: While dairy is a source of vitamin D, you may still need sun exposure or supplements for adequate intake.

Myth: Vitamin D is only important for older adults.

Fact: People of all ages need vitamin D for bone health,

immune function, and overall well-being.

Myth: Vitamin E will prevent scars.

Fact: Vitamin E may support skin healing but doesn't prevent or treat scars.

Myth: All supplements are safe, regardless of dosage.

Fact: Overdosing on vitamins can be dangerous, especially with fat-soluble vitamins like A and D.

Myth: Vitamin B9 (Folate) is only important during pregnancy.

Fact: Folate is crucial for everyone, as it supports DNA repair and cell division.

Myth: Vitamin C can prevent wrinkles.

Fact: Vitamin C supports collagen production but won't directly prevent aging signs like wrinkles.

Myth: You need to take vitamins with a meal for better absorption.

Fact: Some vitamins (like vitamin D) require fat for absorption, while others (like vitamin C) can be taken without food.

Vitamins are essential for maintaining overall health, but there are many myths and misconceptions surrounding them. From the belief that "more is always better" to the idea that all vitamin supplements are created equal, it's important to approach vitamins with an informed mindset. In reality, vitamins should be taken in balanced amounts, tailored to individual needs, and sourced primarily from a healthy, varied diet. Supplements can play a role in addressing specific deficiencies, but they are not a substitute for proper nutrition. Always consult with a healthcare provider before starting new vitamin regimens, and remember: the best way to support your health is through a combination of whole foods, lifestyle practices, and, when necessary, supplements based on scientific guidance. Stay informed, and don't let myths cloud the path to better health!

ΔΔΔ

OPTIMIZE YOUR VITAMINS FASTER

Vitamins play an essential role in maintaining overall health, but the way we store, prepare, and combine our foods can significantly impact their nutritional value. These quick and simple tips can help you optimize the vitamins in your daily meals, ensuring you're getting the most benefit from the food you eat. Whether you're aiming to preserve vitamin content or improve nutrient absorption, these easy steps are designed to help you make small but impactful changes to your routine.

- Store vegetables in dark places to preserve vitamin A
and C content.

-Chop garlic 10 minutes before cooking to activate
vitamin C and other nutrients.

-Steam vegetables instead of boiling to retain
vitamins A and C.

-Eat a rainbow of colors daily to ensure a good balance
of vitamins A, C, D, and E.

-Combine vitamin C-rich foods with iron sources for
better absorption of vitamin C and iron.

-Take vitamin D supplements with fatty meals for
better absorption of fat-soluble vitamins like A, D, and
E.

-Store nuts and seeds in the refrigerator to preserve

vitamin E content.

-Eat local and seasonal fruits and vegetables for the highest vitamin A, C, and E content.

-Include raw foods daily for maximum preservation of vitamin C and E.

-Use the water from steamed vegetables in soups or sauces to capture water-soluble vitamins like C.

-Avoid overcooking vegetables to retain vitamin A, C, and E.

-Add avocado to your salad to boost absorption of fat-soluble vitamins like A, D, and E.

-Drink green tea to improve vitamin C absorption.

-Soak beans overnight to reduce phytic acid, improving mineral and vitamin absorption.

-Pair sweet potatoes with olive oil to boost vitamin A

absorption.

-Use cast iron cookware to increase the iron content in food, supporting vitamin C absorption.

-Take vitamin D supplements with meals for better absorption, especially if you're not getting enough from the sun.

-Include fermented foods like kimchi to support vitamin K absorption, indirectly aiding in vitamin D metabolism.

-Refrigerate fruit juices to preserve vitamin C.

-Consume whole grains for a steady supply of B vitamins, which work synergistically with vitamin E.

-Chew your food thoroughly to ensure better nutrient absorption, including vitamins A, C, and E.

-Add lemon juice to your water to enhance vitamin C intake.

-Avoid excessive alcohol to prevent depletion of vitamin A and D.

-Eat more citrus fruits like oranges and grapefruits for a natural vitamin C boost.

-Blend fruits with a source of fat like avocado or nuts to help absorb fat-soluble vitamins A, D, and E.

-Incorporate leafy greens like spinach and kale for a rich source of vitamins A and C.

-Roast vegetables at lower temperatures to preserve vitamins A and C.

-Use a slow cooker for soups to preserve water-soluble vitamins like C.

-Include almonds, sunflower seeds, or hazelnuts in your diet for vitamin E.

-Keep fruits and vegetables whole until ready to eat to preserve vitamins A, C, and E.

-Sprinkle seeds like chia and flax on your meals for added vitamin E and omega-3s.

-Make smoothies with a variety of fruits for a diverse intake of vitamins A, C, and E.

-Freeze fruits and vegetables shortly after harvest to preserve vitamins, especially C.

-Use a juicer instead of a blender to make vitamin-packed juice with fewer calories, preserving vitamin C.

-Avoid microwaving food as it can degrade vitamin C content.

-Grow your own herbs for a fresh source of vitamin A, C, and E.

-Add turmeric to your meals to enhance the absorption of fat-soluble vitamins like A and E.

-Eat more berries like blueberries and strawberries for

vitamin C.

-Include a variety of cruciferous vegetables like broccoli for vitamins A and C.

-Combine tomatoes with olive oil to improve the absorption of lycopene and vitamin A.

-Consume fish like salmon for a natural vitamin D boost.

-Drink bone broth to support the absorption of fat-soluble vitamins like A and D.

-Squeeze fresh citrus on salads for an extra vitamin C kick.

-Try chia pudding made with almond milk for a vitamin-rich snack, especially vitamin E.

-Cook tomatoes briefly to release more of their vitamin C and lycopene.

-Use fresh herbs like parsley in your cooking to

enhance vitamin C intake.

-Add egg yolks to your meals for a natural source of vitamin D and A.

-Use ginger in smoothies to improve vitamin C absorption.

-Pair vitamin C-rich foods with foods high in bioflavonoids for better absorption.

-Don't discard the skin of fruits and vegetables like apples and carrots for added vitamins A and C.

-Substitute olive oil for butter to enhance the absorption of fat-soluble vitamins A, D, and E.

-Drink water with your meals to help absorption of vitamin C.

-Use flaxseed oil in smoothies to increase vitamin E intake.

-Eat bell peppers for a boost of vitamin C.

-Sprinkle nutritional yeast on popcorn for a B vitamin boost, which works well with vitamin E.

-Soak nuts and seeds overnight to improve nutrient availability and support vitamin E absorption.

-Add dark chocolate to your diet for magnesium and vitamin E.

-Use coconut milk in smoothies for an extra boost of fat-soluble vitamins A and D.

-Use quinoa as a base for salads for added vitamin B and A.

-Roast vegetables with olive oil to enhance vitamin A and E absorption.

-Incorporate mushrooms into your meals for a natural source of vitamin D.

-Drink fortified plant milk for a daily dose of vitamin D and A.

-Top your oatmeal with chia seeds for added vitamin A and E.

-Sprinkle spirulina on salads for a nutrient-dense source of vitamin A and E.

-Add a pinch of black pepper to enhance turmeric's absorption, benefiting vitamin A and E.

-Include more cabbage in your diet for a rich source of vitamin K and vitamin A.

-Use avocado oil in cooking to boost vitamin E intake.

-Drink green smoothies with a protein source to better absorb vitamin D and A.

-Include vitamin C-rich foods like strawberries in your breakfast.

-Drink vegetable-based soups to capture water-soluble vitamins like C.

-Use tahini in salads or wraps for added vitamin E.

-Add a tablespoon of coconut oil to smoothies for better absorption of vitamins A and E.

-Try adding papaya to your diet for a natural source of vitamins A and C.

-Incorporate kale and swiss chard in your meals for a vitamin K and A boost.

-Include a variety of beans in your diet for vitamins and minerals that support overall health.

-Consume vitamin D-rich foods like fortified cereals and eggs regularly.

-Make a green smoothie made with spinach, avocado, and fruit for a vitamin-packed breakfast.

-Use a variety of herbs like basil and cilantro to enhance your vitamin A and C intake.

-Sprinkle hemp seeds on your food for an extra boost of vitamin E and omega-3s.

-Include vitamin E-rich foods like almonds in your daily diet.

-Eat more orange vegetables like carrots and sweet potatoes for vitamin A.

-Drink fresh-pressed juice made from kale, apple, and lemon for vitamins A, C, and E.

-Top your salad with pumpkin seeds for a good source of vitamin E.

-Make smoothies with a variety of fruits for a diverse intake of vitamins A, C, and E.

-Include vitamin A-rich foods like sweet potatoes and carrots in your meals.

-Drink vitamin D-fortified plant milk to support bone health and vitamin D intake.

-Use avocado in your meals for added vitamins A, D, and E.

-Add lemon zest to your smoothie for a boost of vitamin C.

-Top oatmeal with dried apricots for a vitamin A boost.

-Incorporate more leafy greens like arugula for a natural vitamin A and C source.

-Eat vitamin C-rich foods like kiwis and bell peppers with meals to aid iron absorption.

-Pair vitamin C-rich foods with healthy fats to enhance absorption of fat-soluble vitamins A and E.

-Store vegetables in a cool, dark place to preserve vitamin A and C.

-Drink plenty of water to support vitamin C metabolism and absorption.

-Make a fruit salad with strawberries for a vitamin C-packed snack.

-Use olive oil to roast vegetables for better absorption

-Add some citrus zest to your smoothies to increase vitamin C intake.

-Sprinkle ground flaxseed on your meals for a good source of vitamin E.

-Top your salad with bell peppers to enhance your intake of vitamin C.

-Pair broccoli with a squeeze of lemon to maximize vitamin C absorption.

These 100 tips for optimizing vitamins A, C, D, and E are designed to make it easier for you to maximize the nutritional value of the foods you consume. By following simple strategies for food preparation, storage, and combination, you can enhance the absorption and preservation of these essential vitamins in your daily meals. Incorporate these tips into your routine to support your overall health and well-being, ensuring you get the full benefit of your nutrient-packed diet.

$$\triangle\triangle\triangle$$

HISTORICAL WISDOM ON VITAMINS A,C,D AND E

T hroughout history, various cultures around the world have developed unique dietary practices and traditional remedies that unknowingly focused on providing essential vitamins for health. Long before the discovery of vitamins and their role in the human body, ancient civilizations relied on natural sources—be it through specific foods, herbs, or animal products—to maintain vitality and prevent illnesses. From the use of fish oils in Northern cultures to the consumption of citrus in ancient Greece, these practices show a deep understanding of nutrition that transcended time and geography. By examining the rich traditions of different cultures, we can uncover the historical wisdom behind vitamins A, C, D, and E, and learn valuable lessons that can still guide us in optimizing our health today.

Ancient Egypt:

The Egyptians used liver to treat night blindness, unknowingly providing vitamin A. They also applied kohl around their eyes, which helped prevent eye infections—a benefit we now know comes from vitamin A's immune-supporting properties.

Traditional Chinese Medicine:

Chinese healers prescribed sprouted beans for sailors

on long voyages, instinctively understanding these contained vital nutrients (now known to be vitamin C) that prevented scurvy. They also recognized the healing properties of fish oils, rich in vitamins A and D.

Native American Wisdom:

Many Native American tribes dried berries and preserved organ meats, ensuring year-round access to vital nutrients. The Inuit's traditional practice of eating raw liver and fermented fish provided essential vitamins in an environment with limited plant foods.

Mediterranean Traditions:

Greek and Italian cultures traditionally cure olives and incorporate olive oil into daily meals, providing essential vitamin E. Their practice of sun-drying tomatoes actually concentrates vitamin content.

Indian Ayurvedic Practices:

Ayurvedic medicine recommended eating fresh fruits before meals and specific food combinations that we now know enhance vitamin absorption. The traditional practice of exposing milk to sunlight increased its vitamin D content.

Japanese Customs:

The Japanese practice of consuming fermented foods like natto provides vitamin K and other nutrients. Their tradition of eating small portions of raw fish supplies fat-soluble vitamins A and D.

Ancient Greece:

Hippocrates, known as the Father of Medicine,

promoted the use of olive oil for skin health and healing, a rich source of vitamin E, which helps to protect and nourish the skin.

Ancient Rome:

Roman soldiers consumed large amounts of dried figs, a rich source of vitamin C, to protect against scurvy on long military campaigns.

Scandinavian Traditions:

In Nordic countries, traditional diets included fish such as herring and cod, known for their high vitamin D content, helping to prevent rickets in long, dark winters.

Russian Folk Medicine:

Russians used rose hips, a potent natural source of

vitamin C, to treat colds and boost immunity during the harsh winter months.

234

British Colonial Practices:

British sailors were given lemon juice to prevent scurvy, unknowingly consuming large amounts of vitamin C to maintain their health on long voyages.

South American Indigenous Practices:

In the Andes, indigenous people consume foods like quinoa and native potatoes that are rich in antioxidants and vitamin A to support eye health.

African Traditional Remedies:

Various African cultures use baobab fruit, which is loaded with vitamin C, to treat colds and boost the immune system.

French Country Cooking:

French country kitchens have long used egg yolks in dishes like hollandaise sauce, providing a rich source of vitamin D, especially when made with free-range eggs.

Middle Eastern Diet:

In the Middle East, pomegranate is consumed as a fruit rich in vitamin C, historically believed to improve skin health and immune function.

Australian Aboriginal Knowledge:

Aboriginal Australians traditionally consumed bush tomatoes, which are rich in vitamin E, to support skin health and reduce oxidative stress.

Polynesian Practices:

The Polynesians ate large amounts of fish, seaweed, and coconut, providing them with essential vitamins A, D, and E, especially beneficial for bone health.

Chinese Herbal Medicine:

Traditional Chinese healers used herbs like chrysanthemum and goji berries, which are rich in vitamin A, for eye health and anti-aging.

Mexican Cuisine:

The traditional practice of using chili peppers in cooking, especially in dishes like salsa, is not only rich in antioxidants but also in vitamin C, known to support the immune system.

Pacific Northwest Native Practices:

Native American tribes in the Pacific Northwest relied

heavily on salmon and other fatty fish, providing a natural source of vitamin D to combat the long winters.

Portuguese Dietary Traditions:

The Portuguese diet often includes codfish, rich in vitamin D, which helps prevent bone diseases such as rickets and osteoporosis.

Turkish Cuisine:

Turkish traditional cuisine incorporates sunflower seeds, rich in vitamin E, known for their ability to promote heart health and combat free radical damage.

Scandinavian Fermentation:

In Scandinavia, fermented foods like sauerkraut and

pickled herring provide both probiotics and vitamin C, supporting gut health and immunity.

Thai Cooking Traditions:

In Thailand, the use of turmeric in curry dishes is common. Turmeric helps to improve the bioavailability of fat-soluble vitamins like A and E.

Korean Fermentation:

Korean food traditions emphasize fermented vegetables like kimchi, which not only contain probiotic benefits but also provide a rich source of vitamin K.

Hawaiian Traditions:

In Hawaii, the traditional diet includes papaya, rich in vitamin C, which was used by native people to enhance skin health and heal wounds.

Caribbean Healing Practices:

Indigenous Caribbean people used bitter melon, a vegetable rich in vitamin A, to treat diabetes and improve vision health.

Ancient Mesopotamia:

The Sumerians and Babylonians recognized the medicinal properties of certain plants like dates, which are high in vitamin A and C, to support general health and energy.

Native South American Practices:

The Incas consumed the fruit of the acerola cherry, which contains an exceptionally high level of vitamin C, to prevent scurvy and improve immune function.

Ancient Indian Traditions:

In traditional Indian medicine, curry leaves were widely used for their rich vitamin A content to support vision health and general immunity.

Egyptian Honey Use:

Ancient Egyptians applied honey as a wound dressing, and modern studies show honey contains antioxidants that support vitamin E-like activity, promoting skin healing.

Nordic Fish Consumption:

In Nordic cultures, traditional dishes like gravlax (cured salmon) are rich in omega-3 fatty acids and vitamin D, critical for maintaining bone health and immune function.

Southeast Asian Tea:

In countries like Vietnam and Thailand, the leaves of the moringa plant (often called the "drumstick tree") were used in teas to boost vitamin A levels and prevent deficiencies.

Brazilian Indigenous Healing:

The indigenous peoples of Brazil have long used açai berries, rich in vitamin C, as part of their diets to boost immunity and fight oxidative stress.

Mongolian Diet:

The Mongolian diet traditionally consisted of dried meats, which are rich in vitamin D, especially in winter months, helping to maintain bone health during cold seasons.

Inuit Fish Consumption:

Inuit people consume fish like salmon and cod, which are abundant in vitamin D, to support bone health and immune function in the harsh Arctic environment.

South Asian Herbal Practices:

In Ayurveda, herbs like amla (Indian gooseberry) are prized for their high vitamin C content, which is believed to support skin health and boost immunity.

Inuit Seaweed Consumption:

Inuit diets often included seaweed, a rich source of vitamin D and iodine, which are essential for thyroid health and immune function.

Ancient Indian Ghee:

In ancient Indian medicine, ghee (clarified butter) was

used both as a cooking fat and medicinally for its high content of fat-soluble vitamins, particularly vitamin A.

Peruvian Potato Consumption:

In Peru, native potatoes are high in vitamin C, and traditional dishes like "causa" were consumed to prevent scurvy during long winters.

The historical practices and cultural wisdom surrounding vitamins A, C, D, and E highlight the remarkable ways ancient societies nurtured their health through food and natural remedies. Though modern science has provided us with a deeper understanding of the biochemical roles of these vitamins, the traditional knowledge passed down through generations is still relevant today. From the healing properties of fermented fish oils to the vitamin-rich fruits and vegetables that have long supported immune function, these time-tested practices demonstrate how food can be a powerful tool for maintaining wellness. By embracing these traditions, we can enhance our understanding of nutrition and incorporate simple yet effective habits to optimize our vitamin intake and overall health.

ΔΔΔ

BLOW YOUR MIND
WITH VITAMIN FACTS

-Vitamin A is essential for night vision – It helps produce rhodopsin, the pigment responsible for seeing in low light.

-Vitamin D deficiency can lead to weak bones – Without vitamin D, the body struggles to absorb calcium.

-Vitamin C promotes collagen production – It's essential for healthy skin, joints, and tissue repair.

-Vitamin E is a powerful antioxidant – It protects cells from oxidative damage and supports immune health.

-Carrots are packed with vitamin A – They're one of the best natural sources of beta-carotene.

-Vitamin C isn't stored in the body – You need to consume it daily, as excess is excreted.

-Vitamin D enhances calcium absorption – It's crucial for bone health and preventing osteoporosis.

-Vitamin E helps absorb other vitamins – It aids the absorption of vitamins A, D, and K.

-Sunlight provides vitamin D – Just 15-30 minutes in the sun can supply your body with vitamin D.

-Fatty fish like salmon are rich in vitamin D – They're a natural source that supports bone and immune health.

-Vitamin C speeds up wound healing – It's vital for tissue repair and recovery from injuries.

-1 billion people worldwide have vitamin D deficiency

– It's a global health issue, especially in regions with limited sunlight.

-Vitamin A supports immune function – It helps form white blood cells to fight infections.

-Red bell peppers have more vitamin C than oranges – They are one of the richest sources of this nutrient.

-The body makes vitamin D from sunlight – Vitamin D is the only vitamin your body produces naturally from sun exposure.

-Too much vitamin A can be toxic – Excessive intake can cause nausea, dizziness, and even liver damage.

-Vitamin C supports mental health – It plays a role in regulating stress hormones like cortisol.

-Vitamin E can protect against heart disease – It reduces the oxidation of cholesterol, lowering heart disease risk.

-Vitamin C helps fight free radicals – It neutralizes harmful molecules that damage cells.

-Vitamin D is linked to reduced depression – Adequate vitamin D levels help improve mood and well-being.

-Vitamin A is key for healthy skin – It promotes skin cell turnover, reducing wrinkles and acne.

-Vitamin C boosts immunity – It strengthens the immune system and reduces cold symptoms.

-Vitamin D improves muscle strength – It's necessary for muscle function, especially in older adults.

-Vitamin E is crucial for cognitive function – It helps protect brain cells from damage.

-Vitamin C helps with iron absorption – It boosts the absorption of non-heme iron from plant foods.

-Vitamin D helps fight respiratory infections – Adequate levels lower the risk of flu and pneumonia.

-Vitamin A is critical for bone health – It supports the growth and maintenance of bone tissue.

-Vitamin E in nuts reduces inflammation – Almonds and sunflower seeds are great sources of vitamin E.

-Vitamin C may reduce cancer risk – It's a potent antioxidant that helps prevent cell damage.

-Vitamin D helps regulate blood pressure – It may lower the risk of hypertension and heart disease.

-Vitamin A prevents dry eyes – It keeps the eyes moist and prevents conditions like xerophthalmia.

-Vitamin E supports skin health – It helps prevent premature aging and protects against UV damage.

-Vitamin C is key for tissue repair – It helps regenerate damaged skin and supports overall healing.

-Vitamin D can prevent type 2 diabetes – It improves insulin sensitivity and lowers the risk of diabetes.

-Vitamin E helps prevent cataracts – Its antioxidant properties protect eye health and reduce the risk of cataracts.

-Vitamin A supports reproductive health – It's important for both male and female fertility.

-Vitamin C lowers cholesterol levels – It helps reduce LDL cholesterol and improve heart health.

-Vitamin D helps reduce inflammation – It's linked to lower inflammation markers in the body.

-Vitamin A and vitamin D work together – They both help in cell growth and immune system regulation.

-Vitamin E may reduce the risk of Alzheimer's – It helps protect brain cells from oxidative damage.

-Vitamin C boosts energy levels – It reduces fatigue and helps with overall vitality.

-Vitamin D is essential for pregnancy – It supports

fetal development and helps prevent complications.

-Vitamin A promotes healthy teeth – It's important for the development of strong, healthy enamel.

-Vitamin E helps prevent blood clots – It improves circulation and reduces the risk of stroke.

-Vitamin C reduces the severity of colds – It can shorten the duration of symptoms and reduce severity.

-Vitamin D supports healthy pregnancy – Adequate levels help prevent complications like preeclampsia.

-Vitamin A regulates skin cell turnover – It reduces acne and improves skin texture.

-Vitamin C helps with brain function – It supports memory and cognitive performance.

-Vitamin D helps fight chronic disease – Low levels of vitamin D are linked to increased risk of chronic diseases like heart disease.

-Vitamin E promotes heart health – It helps reduce oxidative stress that can damage blood vessels.

-Vitamin A prevents night blindness – It's essential for good vision, especially in low-light conditions.

-Vitamin D promotes healthy teeth – It helps with calcium absorption, improving dental health.

-Vitamin C fights oxidative stress – It reduces the damage caused by free radicals and protects the body.

-Vitamin E helps with wound healing – It supports tissue repair and regeneration.

-Vitamin C is needed for neurotransmitter production – -It's essential for producing serotonin and norepinephrine, which regulate mood.

-Vitamin A supports healthy mucus membranes – It protects the lining of the lungs, gastrointestinal tract, and other organs.

-Vitamin D supports healthy hair growth – It plays a role in the hair follicle cycle, preventing hair loss.

-Vitamin C enhances immune response – It helps white blood cells function more effectively in fighting infections.

-Vitamin A helps with iron absorption – It aids the absorption of iron, particularly in plant-based sources.

-Vitamin D is a mood booster – It's linked to improved mood, reducing symptoms of seasonal affective disorder (SAD).

-Vitamin E reduces the risk of heart attacks – By preventing LDL oxidation, it can lower the likelihood of cardiovascular disease.

-Vitamin C can prevent scurvy – A severe deficiency of

vitamin C causes bleeding gums and skin lesions.

-Vitamin A helps fight infections – It supports the production of immune cells like T-cells and antibodies.

-Vitamin D is essential for bone mineralization – It aids in bone development and helps prevent rickets in children.

-Vitamin E improves blood circulation – It enhances the function of blood vessels and improves overall circulation.

-Vitamin C boosts collagen production – It helps the body produce collagen, essential for skin, joints, and connective tissue.

-Vitamin D helps prevent fractures – Adequate levels improve bone strength, reducing the risk of bone fractures.

-Vitamin A helps in wound healing – It accelerates the repair of damaged tissues.

-Vitamin C protects against skin damage – It shields the skin from UV damage and can reduce signs of aging.

-Vitamin D helps in muscle function – It supports muscle contraction and strength.

-Vitamin A promotes hair growth – It aids in sebum production, keeping the scalp healthy.

-Vitamin E fights skin aging – It protects against oxidative stress and can reduce the appearance of fine lines.

-Vitamin D helps regulate the immune system – It helps activate immune cells to fight off infections.

-Vitamin C prevents oxidative damage – It fights free radicals that can damage cells and lead to chronic disease.

-Vitamin D helps lower the risk of autoimmune diseases – Adequate levels may protect against diseases like multiple sclerosis.

-Vitamin E aids in managing blood sugar – It has potential to help people with diabetes manage their blood glucose levels.

-Vitamin A boosts skin hydration – It promotes the production of sebum, which keeps skin moisturized.

-Vitamin C helps with iron-deficiency anemia – It improves the absorption of iron, especially from plant sources.

-Vitamin D aids in proper cell function – It helps regulate cell growth, repair, and metabolism.

-Vitamin E helps reduce the risk of stroke – It lowers oxidative damage to the blood vessels and arteries.

-Vitamin C aids in detoxification – It supports liver function, helping to flush out toxins from the body.

-Vitamin D helps with sleep – It may help regulate sleep patterns by influencing melatonin production.

-Vitamin E reduces the risk of age-related macular degeneration – It helps protect against vision loss in older adults.

-Vitamin A helps repair the skin – It speeds up skin regeneration and helps heal scars.

-Vitamin C can reduce wrinkles – Its collagen-boosting properties make it a popular ingredient in anti-aging products.

-Vitamin D helps balance hormones – It is important for the production of sex hormones like estrogen and testosterone.

-Vitamin A prevents dry skin – It keeps the skin

moisturized and prevents skin disorders like eczema.

-Vitamin E may help protect against cancer – Its antioxidant properties may lower the risk of certain cancers.

-Vitamin C helps improve gum health – It strengthens gums and prevents gum disease.

-Vitamin D supports the nervous system – It is vital for proper nervous system function.

-Vitamin E promotes hair health – It nourishes the scalp and improves hair growth.

-Vitamin C helps reduce the risk of chronic diseases – It reduces the risk of heart disease and other oxidative stress-related conditions.

-Vitamin D helps prevent high blood pressure – Adequate levels can reduce hypertension risk.

-Vitamin A supports eye health – It helps prevent

vision loss and supports overall eye function.

-Vitamin C enhances iron absorption – It boosts the body's ability to absorb iron from plant-based sources.

-Vitamin D aids in detoxification – It supports the liver's ability to detoxify the body.

-Vitamin E helps with muscle recovery – It reduces muscle soreness and promotes faster recovery after exercise.

-Vitamin C supports overall skin health – It helps protect the skin from damage and promotes a youthful appearance.

-Vitamin D helps manage cholesterol – It helps regulate cholesterol levels and promotes cardiovascular health.

-Vitamin A supports immune system memory – It helps the immune system recognize pathogens and react more effectively.

ΔΔΔ

FINAL THOUGHTS

Our exploration of the world of vitamins reveals an incredible landscape of essential nutrients basic in all spheres of human life. From the fat-soluble vitamins (A, D, E, K) to the water-soluble family (B-complex and C), each vitamin shines out as a unique player in keeping good health with diverse qualities, roles, and challenges in our modern world. The variety and interdependence of these nutrients highlight how well nature supports human health.

Modern living offers heretofore unheard-of challenges for maintaining perfect vitamin status. Indoor life affects vitamin D synthesis; environmental contaminants increase our need for antioxidant defense; and soil depletion affects the nutritional content of our food. Stress, processed foods, and busy lives all further complicate our ability to maintain optimal vitamin levels. These challenges require for cautious preparations to ensure sufficient vitamin consumption and absorption.

Passed down over millennia all around, the cultural understanding of vitamins occasionally precedes scientific knowledge. From Asian tribes fermenting foods high in vitamin C-rich nutrients to Egyptian doctors treating night blindness with liver, ancient methods from numerous civilizations frequently matched what modern science now confirms. Along with contemporary research, this ancient wisdom provides a strong foundation for understanding of vitamin optimization.

Modern research is exposing novel functions for vitamins in human health. Apart from their basic functions, vitamins influence genetic expression, prevent chronic illnesses, and are very vital for sports performance and recovery. In nutritional studies, the connections among vitamins and our microbiota, their roles in mental health, and their influence on aging processes provide interesting new approaches.

Age, lifestyle, genetic makeup, and environmental exposures all affect individual vitamin needs somewhat differently. While food sources often provide better absorption and usage, targeted supplements can be quite beneficial in handling modern nutritional problems. Understanding these special variations helps to develop more effective plans for optimizing vitamins.

Looking ahead, emerging technologies provide more accurate ways to monitor and maximize vitamin status. Customized techniques based on environmental exposure assessment, genetic testing, and individual health goals may produce more successful vitamin optimization regimens. Resilience and health depend more on maintaining appropriate vitamin status as we negotiate changing lifestyles and environmental issues.

Success with vitamins requires understanding their complex roles and interactions in human health rather than reliance solely on simple supplementation. Although preventing deficiency is still important, increasing vitamin status for best performance and long-term health is a more all-encompassing goal. Together with reasonable application strategies, this understanding helps to create effective ways for maintaining optimal vitamin status in our modern world.

[Final Insight: As we keep finding new functions and interactions for vitamins in human health, their importance in adapting to present challenges becomes more clear. Maintaining health and vitality in our changed environment depends mostly on intentional optimization of vitamin level.]

△△△

BOOKS BY THIS AUTHOR

9 Golden Rules Of Nutrition

Unlock the secrets to a healthier you with "9 Golden Rules of Nutrition"

Are you tired of complicated diet plans and confusing nutritional advice? Look no further! This easy-to-follow guide will revolutionize the way you think about food and nourishment.

In this concise and powerful ebook, you'll discover:

• 9 simple yet effective rules to transform your eating habits
• Clear explanations that anyone can understand
• Practical tips for implementing these rules in your daily life

Say goodbye to fad diets and hello to sustainable, long-term health. Whether you're a busy professional, a parent juggling multiple responsibilities, or someone who wants to improve their well-being, this book is for you.

Inside, you'll learn:

1. How to balance your plate for optimal nutrition
2. The truth about portion sizes and how to control them effortlessly
3. Why hydration is crucial and how to ensure you're drinking enough
4. The power of whole foods and how to incorporate them into your meals
5. Smart strategies for reducing sugar and processed food intake
6. The importance of mindful eating and how it can change your relationship with food
7. How to make healthier choices when dining out or on-the-go
8. Tips for meal planning and preparation to set yourself up for success

Each golden rule is explained in simple terms, making it easy to grasp and apply the concepts immediately. There is no more confusion or overwhelm—just straightforward, actionable advice.

But this book isn't just about rules. It's about empowering you to make informed decisions about your health. You'll gain a deeper understanding of how food affects your body and mind, allowing you to take control of your well-being.

The best part? These rules are flexible and adaptable

to any lifestyle. Whether you're a vegetarian, follow a specific dietary restriction, or want to eat better, you'll find valuable insights that work for you.

Imagine waking up each day feeling energized, focused, and ready to tackle whatever comes your way. Picture yourself effortlessly making healthier choices without feeling deprived or restricted. That's the power of these 9 golden rules.

This ebook is perfect for:

• Beginners who are just starting their health journey
• Those who have tried countless diets with little success
• Anyone looking to simplify their approach to nutrition
• People who want to improve their overall health and well-being
• Parents seeking to instill healthy habits in their children

Don't waste another day feeling confused about what to eat. With "9 Golden Rules of Nutrition," you'll have a clear roadmap to better health right at your fingertips.

Ready to transform your relationship with food and take charge of your health? Grab your copy now and start your journey towards a happier, healthier you!

Remember, good nutrition doesn't have to be complicated. Let these 9 golden rules guide you to a life of vitality and wellness. Your body will thank you!